HOMEOPATHY
for
MENOPAUSE

*H*OMEOPATHY
for
*M*ENOPAUSE

BETH MacEOIN

Healing Arts Press
Rochester, Vermont

*This book is dedicated to Morris,
with all my love.*

Healing Arts Press
One Park Street
Rochester, Vermont 05767
www.gotoit.com

Note to the reader: This book is intended as an informational guide. The remedies, approaches, and techniques described herein are meant to supplement, and not to be a substitute for, professional medical care or treatment. They should not be used to treat a serious ailment without prior consultation with a qualified health care professional.

LIBRARY OF CONGRESS CATALOGING-IN-PUBLICATION DATA
MacEoin, Beth.
    Homeopathy for menopause / Beth MacEoin
    p.   cm.
    Includes bibliographical references and index.
    ISBN 0-89281-648-1 (alk. paper)
    1. Menopause—Complications—Homeopathic treatment. 2. Menopause—
Popular works. I. Title.
    RX469.M33 1997
    618.1'7506—dc21   97-6962
                                               CIP

Printed and bound in Canada

10 9 8 7 6 5 4 3 2

This book was typeset in M Bembo

Healing Arts Press is a division of Inner Traditions International

~

Contents

~

~

Acknowledgments

Many thanks are due to the following, for the help and advice they have given during the writing of this book. They include Teresa Chris, Sato Liu, Dr. Andrew Lockie, Jane Graham-Maw, Wanda Whiteley, Natalia Link, and Emma Waghorn. Denis, Jonathan, and Daniel must be thanked for the encouragement and patient support they have given on practical, as well as emotional levels. Many thanks are also due to my mother Nancy, for being there.

~

Foreword

Menopause was once regarded as a time for women to develop the full potential of their lives, for experience and wisdom were highly valued. During the nineteenth century, however, a very different view of the older woman began to emerge. The Victorian gynecologist Edward Tilt saw menopause as "a gradual loss of feminine grace," leading to erratic behavior, melancholia, kleptomania, alcoholism, and even suicide.

As well as espousing the views of Tilt, the American gynecologist Robert Wilson, writing in a medical journal in 1963, warned "the unpalatable truth must be faced that all post-menopausal women are castrates." Later he wrote, "The unwholesome effects of this disease include . . . ugly body contours, flaccidity of the breasts, and atrophy of the genitalia." Administer estrogen to such women, he asserted, "and they become much more pleasant to live with and will not become dull and unattractive."

Unfortunately such views continue to cloud popular opinion. The Amarant Trust, a British pro-HRT (Hormone Replacement Therapy) campaigning organization, asserts in its literature that HRT can stop women from becoming "seriously forgetful" in their old age. "Institutions are full of old women who have become virtual cabbages due to senile decay (Alzheimer's disease), which afflicts more women than men." A scare tactic if ever there was one! This claim has in fact been disputed by American medical researchers.

After a century of such negative conditioning, no wonder a great many women dread the onset of menopause as if it were the beginning of a gray avenue of physical and mental deterioration, heightened by the loss of their fertility and hence, their worth as women. The truth is, very few women experience *every* physical and emotional symptom associated with this transitional phase. Moreover, a great many pass through the change of life with little or no discomfort at all, though for obvious reasons doctors rarely get to hear of such women. As Beth MacEoin so rightly says, there is life after menopause.

Nevertheless, it would be wrong to conclude that all menopausal symptoms are caused by our negative attitudes to aging. Body and mind are inseparably linked, so natural hormonal changes are bound to cause a certain degree of physical and emotional discomfort, at least for a year or so, until everything settles down.

In my own experience as a holistic practitioner, women who have undergone a radical hysterectomy (involving removal of the ovaries) tend to do well on HRT. The same cannot be said for healthy women experiencing a natural menopause. Despite tireless campaigns by doctors and the drug companies, the niggling side effects of HRT can be so distressing that half of all women prescribed the drug stop within six months, according to a recent survey by the National Opinion Polls (U.K.). Clearly, the "feel good" drug is not living up to its expectations.

However, as you are about to discover, there is a gentle alternative in the guise of homeopathy. This system of healing can be of enormous benefit to those suffering physical and emotional symptoms triggered by menopause. The beauty of homeopathy is that the remedies are highly potent and yet completely free of the toxic side effects associated with conventional drug therapy. As the author explains, when chosen and administered correctly, a homoeopathic remedy acts in the manner of a catalyst, gently stimulating the mind-body's innate self-healing processes. Indeed, the benefits can be remarkable, and I can testify to this.

What is refreshingly different about this manual is that the author takes a much broader perspective than the average homeopath. She extols the virtues of such things as deep breathing, conscious relaxation, aromatic bathing, and a whole-food diet to promote good health and a sense of well-being. By taking her advice, we create within our whole being an environment conducive to the efficacy of homeopathic treatment—and indeed, any other therapy we may wish to embark upon.

I encourage you to read this book and to experience for yourself the remarkable healing powers of homeopathic remedies, thus enabling you to positively sail through the autumn of your life.

Chrissie Wildwood
Aromatherapy and Flower Remedy Consultant
September 1995

~

Introduction

It is becoming increasingly obvious that the subject of menopause
has at last come out of the closet. Growing numbers of women are
making it abundantly clear that there is life after menopause. They
are also pointing out that the emotional and physical transforma-
tions that inevitably occur during and after this major watershed
need not involve a change for the worse. In many instances they
may even bring an unexpected change for the better.

Many women report an increased dynamism and a sense of
direction in the years following menopause. As domestic commit-
ments decrease or change, they discover that they have time to ful-
fil their own needs and interests. However, this positive outcome is
often dependent on having enough information to prepare for the
challenge ahead. As with any other major life event, we can eliminate much of the fear that menopause elicits if we are aware of the
options available to us. We can then take positive steps to ensure
that we actively support our experience of menopause, rather than
fruitlessly denying it at every step. We do not have to accept that
we have suddenly become old crones; many of us will still have as
much interest in how we look and feel about ourselves as we did in
our thirties. However, accepting the physical and emotional matu-
rity that comes with menopausal and postmenopausal years is a vital
part of this transition.

By becoming more familiar with our overall state of health and the working of our bodies, we can take the first step on this bewildering, daunting, but ultimately exciting journey.

WHAT IS MENOPAUSE?

Strictly speaking, menopause occurs when we have our last menstrual period. The average age for this is around fifty, but many of us will have experienced a range of symptoms for years before menopause occurs.

Such symptoms include changes in our monthly cycles, with periods becoming irregular, shorter, longer, scantier, or much heavier. If we normally suffer from premenstrual syndrome, symptoms may become more severe, or we may find that we are beginning to experience hot flashes or night sweats. Mood swings, forgetfulness, anxiety, and bouts of depression may also occur. Leading up to menopause, our periods may gradually taper off before they disappear altogether, or they may stop more abruptly. Because of the difficulty in establishing when menopause has occurred, it is wise to continue using contraceptive measures for a year or two after the last period. Other symptoms that may occur during the premenopausal years include headaches, migraines, low libido, sleep disturbance, itchy skin, and vaginal dryness and itching.

Although the average age for experiencing menopause is fifty, some women may stop menstruating around the age of forty-five, while others may continue until they are mid-way through their fifties. An earlier than average menopause may occur at any time between thirty-five and forty-five, and in exceptional circumstances, a premature menopause may occur before the age of thirty-five. Factors that would result in an early menopause include the following:

- removal of the ovaries during a surgical procedure such as hysterectomy;

- radiotherapy;
- diseases that involve an autoimmune reaction, where the body begins to attack its own tissues.

Examples of autoimmune diseases include rheumatoid arthritis and lupus. Although not an autoimmune disease, mumps may also damage the ovaries in rare instances. Other factors that may hasten an earlier onset of menopausal symptoms include a lower than average body weight, cigarette smoking, and a poor-quality diet that is low in essential nutrients.

Once we have entered a postmenopausal phase, we may experience the following symptoms: painful intercourse due to increased dryness of the vagina, genital irritation as a result of thinning vaginal walls, frequent urge to urinate, stress incontinence, and dryness of the skin and hair. Later symptoms may include general aches and pains, thinning bones, and circulatory problems.

SEVERITY OF SYMPTOMS

Although the lists given above make rather sobering reading, it is apparent that, although some of us may experience a range of distressing symptoms during these years, others appear to sail through menopause with comparatively little distress. Certain factors have been identified as possibly contributing to a more traumatic experience of menopause and the years immediately before and after it. These include:

- an early menopause;
- a history of painful periods;
- long-standing, severe symptoms of premenstrual syndrome;
- low body weight;
- early marriage and early pregnancy.

Factors that may lead to a less distressing menopausal experience include the following:

- late marriage and late pregnancy or remaining unmarried or childless;
- being well-educated and/or financially secure;
- beginning periods at a late age;
- average or above average body weight.

STRATEGIES FOR COPING

Once we are prepared for the problems we are likely to encounter, we can begin to work out how we will choose to support ourselves through this vital transition. We will find that we have a number of options open to us. These include conventional and alternative medical approaches.

The Conventional Medical Approach

This is the avenue that many of us will naturally explore first, since it is likely to be the medical system that we have accepted as the norm since childhood. Treatments for menopausal problems usually include drugs that suppress symptoms such as vaginal or bladder infections, or hormone therapy that seeks to supplement waning supplies of female hormones. The latter may be supplied in the form of patches, tablets, implants, or creams. Psychological and emotional symptoms may be treated with drugs, such as antidepressants and tranquilizers, or with psychotherapy and counseling. Screening is also used to check that certain health problems have not developed, such as osteoporosis (brittle bones) or breast tumors.

The Alternative Medical Approach

A growing number of patients are seeking a different approach to medical treatment, feeling that conventional perspectives are unsuited to their needs. This includes many women who are approaching or experiencing menopause. They may have already tried conventional medication and found it inappropriate or unsatisfactory. These are often women who are attracted by the holistic perspective of alternative approaches with their emphasis on treating the whole person on mental, emotional, and physical levels. Treatment is tailored to each individual with the aim of restoring the optimum balance between mind, emotions, and body. This approach is especially well suited to menopausal conditions, which span a broad range of physical and emotional problems. It is also very attractive to the woman who wants to take an active role in managing her health and improving overall vitality, since she is likely to be encouraged to improve her lifestyle. This may involve adopting a more nutritious eating plan, exercising more, or learning how to relax. In any event, feeling that we can take positive, dynamic action at this time can be an essential factor in transforming menopause into an empowering experience.

In reality, many women will opt for a compromise between conventional and alternative approaches. They may monitor their general state of health through regular checkups and screening procedures available through their GP. However, if they become unhappy about long-term drug use or the unacceptable side effects that are often associated with conventional medicines, they are increasingly likely to choose alternative systems of treatment, such as homeopathy, herbal medicine, or acupuncture, for any problems that emerge.

Introduction

HOMEOPATHY AND MENOPAUSE

Homeopathy is a system of healing that is especially appropriate for treating many of the problems that arise before, during and after menopause. Because the whole person is treated rather than isolated groups of symptoms, emotional problems are given as much weight as physical ones. When healing takes place, the patient feels better on all levels. As a result, a reduction of symptoms such as hot flashes, heavy periods, or insomnia should be accompanied by a measurable boost in energy levels and a sense of enhanced well-being.

Because this improved state is achieved by stimulation of the body's self-regulating mechanism, once this process has begun, further medication is unnecessary unless symptoms return later on. As a result, successful homeopathic treatment offers the exciting prospect of a holistic therapy without the long-term use of medication and without distressing side effects.

Homeopathic treatment is appropriate for a wide range of menopausal problems, which are discussed in the later chapters of this book. Along with a description of each condition, you will find advice on whether the problem is appropriate for home prescribing or whether you need to seek professional help. In addition, basic information is given about general changes in lifestyle you can make that will promote an overall improvement.

1

Homeopathy for Beginners

If you are a newcomer to homeopathy, this chapter will give you the basic information you need to understand the homeopathic perspective on health and healing.

THE BASICS: GENERAL BACKGROUND

Homeopathic medicine has been in existence for around two hundred years. The founder of homeopathic medicine, Samuel Hahnemann, developed a radical, alternative system of healing, which directly challenged the popular, orthodox medical views of his day. Today, professional and medically trained homeopaths treat patients for a range of medical problems on a worldwide scale. Homeopathy is particularly well established in Britain, India, Germany, France, and the Netherlands. It is also gaining ground in South America, the United States, and Eastern Europe.

HISTORICAL BACKGROUND

Samuel Hahnemann was born in Meissen, Germany, in 1755. Although a gifted linguist, he chose to pursue a career in medicine and qualified as a doctor in 1779. Because of the distressing side effects that resulted from popular conventional treatments of that time, Hahnemann decided to abandon his career as an orthodox physician in 1796. He pursued a new career of translating foreign medical texts, while he conducted experiments into gentler ways of restoring sick patients to health.

Hahnemann made a major discovery as a result of translating Cullen's *Materia Medica* (1790). In this text, Cullen suggested that cinchona bark was an effective treatment for the symptoms of malaria because of its astringent properties. Hahnemann, however, was not satisfied with Cullen's reasoning and decided to conduct some research of his own, in search of a more persuasive answer. This involved taking regular doses of cinchona bark and recording its effects. Hahnemann was fascinated by the results yielded by this experiment, since he discovered that while he took cinchona bark he experienced malaria symptoms. Once he stopped taking it, the symptoms subsided. This discovery proved to be the cornerstone of Hahnemann's new system of healing, which he called homeopathy. This involves treating patients with "similar medicines" rather than those that act by opposing disease. Similar medicines can stimulate the healing process when given to someone whose disease symptoms resemble those that are triggered when the same substance is given to a healthy person. As a result of this insight, Hahnemann was to go on developing the theory and practice of homeopathy until his death in Paris in 1843.

As Hahnemann developed and refined his ideas, he came to the conclusion that the functions of the human body are governed by a basic intelligence, or "vital force," which maintains the state of balance and harmony we associate with good health. If this vital force comes into conflict with a stressful stimulus that overloads it, symptoms of ill health will follow. From this perspective, symptoms can be seen in a positive light, since they are signs of the body's incomplete attempts to rid itself of illness. As a result, they can provide us with vital clues to the nature of the problem and give us the essential information on which to base the selection of an appropriate homeopathic remedy.

BASIC PRINCIPLES

There are certain essential concepts that make homeopathy radically different from orthodox medicine. These include:

- the concept of similars;
- the single dose;
- the minimum dose;
- the importance of treating the whole person.

The Concept of Similars

Homeopathic medicines, unlike conventional drugs, are chosen on the basis of the similarity of their effects to the symptoms of illness. For example, if someone experienced an abrupt, violent onset of high fever, restlessness, irritability, and dry, red skin, with sensitivity to bright light, noise, and movement, a homeopath is likely to choose Belladonna as the appropriate remedy. This is because the symptoms listed are identical to those of Belladonna poisoning.

By giving a homeopathic preparation of Belladonna to someone who suffers from these symptoms, homeopaths believe that the body responds to the stimulus of the similar remedy by throwing off the symptoms of illness. In other words, instead of neutralizing the symptoms by opposing them, homeopathic medicines work by activating the body's self-healing mechanism. As a result, once this process is well underway, the remedy has done all that is required, and no further stimulation is needed.

This situation provides a sharp contrast to the prescription of conventional drugs, which are usually given for an extended period, usually on a daily basis. Orthodox drugs act by suppressing or opposing symptoms, instead of supporting the body in its efforts to come to terms with the illness itself. As a result, these drugs can only hold symptoms down for a limited period; once that is over, additional doses of these drugs are usually given in order to maintain the status quo.

The Single Dose

Although it is possible to buy combination preparations of homeopathic medicines for specific problems such as hay fever or travel sickness, it is most usual for homeopaths to prescribe a single remedy at a time. Once this is done, reactions to the medicine's action will be observed, and the decision will be taken by the practitioner whether to wait, repeat a second dose of the same remedy, or change the prescription altogether. This judgment will be made by assessing how fundamental an improvement has been made to the patient's overall condition on all levels. As you can imagine, if multiple remedies are given at any one time, it is almost impossible to know which positive reactions relate to which remedy. As a result, it would be very difficult to decide which of these medicines needs to be repeated.

One of the major reasons for giving a single remedy at a time is linked to the way information has been gathered about each homeopathic medicine. This material can be obtained from accounts of poisonings or as a result of a homeopathic "proving." Proving is a procedure in which a group of volunteers agrees to take regular doses of a substance over an extended period. In order for the proving to render the most accurate information about the medicinal substance, the provers must be in a good state of health and ready to note any changes that occur during the experiment on mental, emotional, or physical levels. The detailed information that comes from the proving is then analyzed, and the symptoms that occurred during the experiment are graded according to their frequency and strength.

Because there has been a tradition of conducting provings with single substances, information is not reliably available about the effects of combination remedies. Therefore, many homeopaths are happier to work with single doses of remedies, about which they have detailed and well-documented material available. However, there are occasional situations where a combination formula might be of use. This would include the rare situations where it is very difficult to differentiate between the relevant remedies needed, such as in an acute case of travel sickness or hay fever. On the other hand, it must be emphasized that these preparations will only give temporary relief: for more profound results to occur, it is necessary to seek more deep-acting, "constitutional" treatment from a homeopathic practitioner.

The Minimum Dose

Hahnemann was adamant that the patient should be given the medicine in the smallest dose required to stimulate a cure. This preoccupation of Hahnemann's dates from the time he spent in practice as a conventional doctor, when he was distressed and appalled by the side effects he witnessed in patients who were given large doses of orthodox drugs.

In many cases, the conventional treatments considered effective at that time gave rise to symptoms that were far worse than those of the original disease. It was common practice for physicians to prescribe large doses of mercury for syphilis, calomel (mercurous chloride) for the many conditions that were thought to require purging, and bleeding or cupping for inflammatory problems. The more Hahnemann witnessed the severely weakened state of these patients, the more convinced he became that there must be a gentler and more effective way to restore a sick person to health.

As a result, he began to experiment with "similar" medicines (*see* "The Concept of Similars," p. 3) in an effort to make the patient's experience less traumatic. As he worked with these medicines, he discovered that they still produced some side effects, and so he began to reduce the dose by diluting them with water. He continued to increase the dilution until he reached the point where no molecules of the original medicine could possibly remain. To everyone's surprise, instead of having a weaker action, these incredibly dilute remedies had a more powerful curative effect on the patient, provided they had also gone through a process of vigorous shaking or pounding, known as *succussion*, and the symptoms of the remedy matched the patient's symptoms as closely as possible.

The Importance of Treating the Whole Person

One of the most important features of homeopathic medicine is its emphasis on treating people rather than diseases. Orthodox medicine stresses the importance of identifying the disease agent and combating the problem with drugs or surgery. A homeopathic approach, on the other hand, emphasizes that it is the body's self-healing mechanism that must be supported, so that illness can be overcome by the body's own efforts. As a result, it is immaterial whether the problem is bacterial or viral in nature, since our immune systems are equipped to fight both perfectly efficiently, provided we remain in good health.

From a homeopathic perspective, the remedy that has the greatest potential for stimulating self-healing must be the one with effects that match the overall symptom "picture" of the patient as a whole. If the correspondence between the selected remedy and symptoms of illness is as great as possible, a homeopathic medicine acts as a catalyst, providing the energy boost that is needed to kick our defence mechanisms into more efficient action.

In order to grasp the idea of this symptom "picture," we need to consider the information about illness that is relevant to a homeopath. Unlike conventional doctors, who stress the impor-

tance of common symptoms in the pursuit of a diagnosis, homeopaths are far more interested in symptoms that convey a sense of
individuality about the patient and his or her symptoms. If we
take the most straightforward example of influenza, common
symptoms associated with this condition include feverishness,
aching limbs, shivering, general prostration, sore throat, and nasal
congestion, and there may be additional complications such as a
cough or inflammation of the sinuses. While this information is
helpful in suggesting the likely diagnosis of flu, it will not help
anyone to identify the most appropriate homeopathic remedy.
A homeopath will ask questions about the speed of onset of the
illness, the nature of nasal discharges, body temperature, the
amount of perspiration, the level of appetite and thirst, any characteristic features of the cough, and any emotional changes since
the illness began.

Once these questions have been answered, we may find that,
although two people are suffering from the same condition, each
person experiences the problem in a unique way. For example,
one flu sufferer may complain of having felt unwell for several
days, with chills and shivers running up and down the spine,
violent sneezing, a severe, slow-developing headache with a
bandlike feeling around the forehead, dizziness, heavy, drooping
eyelids, total apathy and weakness, sweatiness, dark red face
when feverish, and a tendency to be very withdrawn and
depressed since the illness developed. Another person suffering
from the same problem may experience a rapid, violent onset of
symptoms with a dramatic rise in temperature. Severe headaches
or earaches may develop quickly with high temperature, hot,
burning skin, a dry, tickly throat, extreme restlessness and fear
with high fever, and a tendency to panic because of physical discomfort. All these symptoms may be worse at night and may
develop rapidly after severe emotional trauma, shock, or exposure to extreme chill or cold winds. As we can see from these
two examples, although there are certain common features,

7

there are enough differentiating characteristics on which to base a homeopathic prescription. As a result, Gelsemium would be an appropriate homeopathic remedy for the first patient, and Aconite for the second.

We can apply the same principle of searching for these individualizing characteristics whenever we are attempting to select the most appropriate remedy. This is what we constantly have to bear in mind when we are attempting to find the most suitable remedy for any condition, from hot flashes to insomnia.

2

Practical Information:
How to Use This Book to Maximum Advantage

In this chapter you will find all the practical information you are likely to need when you initially explore the possibilities of homeopathy for yourself. As a beginner, there will be numerous basic questions you are likely to ask. If they are not answered in this section, they will be covered by the books included in the general reading lists given at the back of the book. Start gradually, building up your confidence over time and only tackling those situations you feel at ease with. You will be surprised at how empowering and rewarding it can be to take a proactive role in managing your overall health and well-being.

HOW TO BEGIN:
LISTING THE SYMPTOMS

Make a list of the symptoms that have occurred since the onset of your problem. Remember that you are interested in symptoms that represent a change from your normal state, such as the onset of lethargy or fatigue if you are usually full of energy, or chilliness if you are normally warm.

Make the list as complete as possible, including symptoms that may affect you on physical and emotional levels. Even though you may be most concerned about a physical symptom, if you have experienced an emotional reaction since the problem began, this too is extremely important.

By now you should have a list of symptoms that can be arranged in separate sections. The first category should be "typical features." Symptoms that come under this heading should be characteristic of the problem: for example, a factor common to all the symptoms such as burning or dryness. Under this heading you could also make a note of any precipitating factor that occurred before symptoms set in, such as emotional shock or strain.

The second heading will be "general symptoms." Here you can list in detail any changes in your physical and mental well-being since illness began. It may strike you as you are putting this section together that certain features run through your symptoms as a theme or thread, such as dryness, itchiness, or sluggishness. You may also become aware that you have a symptom that is unusual, such as dry mouth without thirst or burning pains that are eased when heat is applied or hot drinks taken. Homeopaths refer to these as rare, strange, and peculiar symptoms, and regard them as extremely important, since they can often clinch a choice of remedy.

You will probably find that the information in the general symptoms list overlaps with that in the typical features list. This is fine, but it is important that the details you list under general symptoms expand the overall symptom picture.

Last of all, you need to list the factors that make you feel better or worse. Remember that this does not just refer to the things that make your specific symptoms improve or not, but those features that make you *generally* better or worse.

You are now ready to consult the relevant table, initially glancing down the typical features list to see which one matches most closely the information in your own first column. If you feel you have found a close enough match, you can consider the information given in the general symptoms section to see if this also fits your symptom picture. Remember, you are unlikely to be presented with a perfect match; what you are looking for is a broad correspondence between your symptoms and the information in the relevant section of the table. If you are happy that the information in the "better for" and "worse from" columns confirms your selection, the chances are that the homeopathic remedy suggested in the last column will be an appropriate first choice.

If at this stage you feel you need further information on which to base your selection of an appropriate remedy, or to confirm your current decision, turn to chapter 7, which provides a check list of homeopathic remedies. Here you will find additional information about each homeopathic medicine, summing up the essential features.

Remember that you do not have to self-prescribe if you feel you are not ready to do so. You may be more at ease with initially using the information in the practical self-help sections, while you familiarize yourself with some of the most commonly used homeopathic medicines and some basic homeopathic theory. How we build up our knowledge and experience of homeopathy depends very much on our individual personalities: some of us will be very eager to have "hands-on," practical experience as quickly as possible and will learn about the theory behind homeopathic prescribing as we go along. Others may feel much more at ease if they spend some time expanding their knowledge about the theory and practice of homeopathic medicine before they are ready to self-prescribe. Take things at your own pace, and never feel obliged to take on anything you feel ill-equipped or unhappy to deal with.

HOW TO TAKE HOMEOPATHIC MEDICINES

Once you have selected a homeopathic remedy that you are confident fits your symptoms well, tip out a single tablet on to a clean spoon or the lid of the remedy bottle. To avoid contamination, it is best not to handle the tablets. If they should spill accidentally, always throw them out rather than replacing them in the bottle.

Avoid taking your remedy too soon after eating when you may still have strong flavors in your mouth. This also applies to eating sweets, having a cup of tea, or cleaning your teeth. Always chew or suck your tablet so that the remedy is absorbed through the mucous membranes of the mouth, rather than swallowing it down with a glass of water.

If your remedies are stored in a dark, cool (but not as cold as the fridge) and reasonably odor-free environment, they should have an indefinite shelf-life. Always replace the cap firmly on the bottle, and never leave the tablets exposed to strong or direct sunlight.

There are certain substances that are thought to interfere with the action of homeopathic medicines. These include strong tea, coffee, peppermint, camphor rubs, and some essential oils such as eucalyptus, rosemary, lavender, and thyme. If you are a newcomer to homeopathic prescribing, it is best to avoid these substances so that your selected remedy has the best chance of working. If you are being treated by a homeopathic practitioner, he or she is also likely to suggest that you avoid contact with these substances.

Dosage

After you have taken your first dose, wait and observe any reaction that takes place. If you experience an initial improvement that relapses after a few hours, you should repeat the remedy. You can proceed along these lines for a day or two until the symptoms clear completely.

If you experience an improvement that holds, you do not need to repeat the dosage, since this is a sign that self-healing has begun and no further stimulation is needed unless, and until, the symptoms return.

If there is little response after taking your remedy, and you are still confident about your choice, repeat the dose and wait to see if an improvement takes place. If a remedy initially helps, but you need to repeat it frequently to maintain an improvement, or if it stops helping, you may need to take the same remedy in a higher potency.

If you initially respond well to your selected remedy, but your symptoms change, you need to go back to the relevant table and check to see if another remedy is more strongly indicated.

An improvement in overall well-being with a short-lived intensification of your original symptoms can often be an indication that you have repeated your remedy over too long a period or too frequently. If this is the case, once you stop taking the remedy, you should find that an improvement sets in rapidly and decisively. This is because too much stimulation has been given too quickly, and an overreaction has taken place. This is quite different from a situation where the symptoms are getting worse of their own accord. If you suspect the latter is true, you should seek professional advice.

Remember that homeopathic medicines are designed to be taken on a short-term basis only. If you find you are needing to repeat your selected remedy on a regular or long-term basis to maintain an improvement, it is important to seek professional help. This is because your reaction would suggest that the remedy (or the potency) you have been taking is not dealing with the problem at a sufficiently deep level to resolve the situation. A homeopath will be trained to stand back from your case and analyze the information objectively, taking into account your full medical and family history as well as a detailed account of your physical, emotional, and mental state. Whatever homeopathic prescription is made will be designed to stimulate your body's capacity for self-healing. Once this process has been activated, you do not need any further homeopathic help unless, and until, your problems return.

If you are in any doubt about your symptoms, or you are concerned that self-help measures are not helping sufficiently with your problem, do not be afraid to seek professional advice. This may come from an orthodox or alternative medical source, depending on the urgency and severity of the condition. It is always safest to err on the cautious side where your health is at stake.

A NOTE ON POTENCIES

Most health food shops and pharmacies will stock homeopathic medicines in a 6c or 30c potency. The *c* stands for the centessimal scale of dilution. To make a homeopathic medicine in a 1c potency, the original substance that is to be made into a remedy must be rendered soluble. This may be done by immersing plants in an alcohol solution or by grinding more resistant matter, such as metals or other minerals, with a pestle and mortar, until it can also be made soluble in a liquid suspension. One drop of this solution is added to ninety-nine drops of alcohol and shaken vigorously to give us our remedy in a 1c potency. A single drop of this potency is then added to ninety-nine drops of alcohol. Once this has also been shaken the required number of times, we have the next potency: 2c. This process can continue until infinitesimal dilutions are reached and no molecules of the original substance are left in the solution. Recent research suggests that, when dilution and succussion take place, the water and alcohol base acts as a polymer or plastic, which takes the imprint of the original molecular structure, transforming it into a substance that has a dynamic potential.

You may also come across homeopathic remedies that have a *d* or *x* on the label. These have gone through a similar process of dilution, but nine drops of alcohol are used each time, instead of ninety-nine. Remedies made in this way belong to the decimal scale.

It is important to remember that potency does not decrease with dilution, it *increases*. The process of dilution and succussion make the remedy more potent, and the higher the potency the more powerful is the effect of the remedy (provided it matches the symptoms of the patient).

HOW TO START: THE POTENCIES TO BUY

As a newcomer to homeopathic prescribing, you will probably find remedies in the 6c potency adequate for your needs. By building up a basic selection of remedies in this way, you can consider adding remedies in the 12c or 30c potencies to your kit at a later stage. As a home prescriber, it is best to limit yourself to remedies of no more than 30c potency. A basic principle of homeopathy is that the gentlest stimulation possible should be given to effect a cure. It is important to be aware that, even though homeopathic medicines can stimulate a cumulative and gentle cure in experienced hands, they are also extremely powerful and dynamic medicines that need to be treated with respect. The higher potencies (200c, 1M, 10M, and beyond) are therefore best used by professionals rather than beginners.

DECIDING WHICH POTENCY TO GIVE, AND HOW OFTEN

As a rule, if symptoms are of recent onset and reasonably mild in nature, it is appropriate to begin the suitable remedy in a 6c potency. The dose may be repeated every hour or two until symptoms improve if the problem is acute, or two to three times a day for a couple of days if the symptoms are more established. If partial relief is obtained using the 6c potency, but symptoms return once the remedy is withdrawn, you should move on to the same remedy in a 12c or 30c potency, remembering that these will require less frequent repetition because they are higher potencies. If you are confident about your choice of remedy, do not worry unduly about the potency, but use what you have to hand. In other words, if all you have is a 6c, but you feel a higher potency is indicated, take the 6c anyway, and you may be surprised at the results.

WHERE TO BUY YOUR HOMEOPATHIC MEDICINES

Homeopathic medicines are becoming increasingly easy to obtain from pharmacies and health food shops. Although these outlets may be appropriate to your needs when you begin, you are likely to find that the range of remedies and potencies they supply are too limited as you become more adventurous in your prescribing. If you are concerned about product reliability, you should contact one of the homeopathic pharmacies or suppliers that specialize in producing and dispensing homeopathic remedies. This is often the best source for obtaining homeopathic medicines since the staff is usually trained to give practical help and advice to those who are new to homeopathy. You may order by mail or telephone if you do not have a homeopathic pharmacy near you. For a list of suppliers see the resources section at the back of the book.

SUGGESTED REMEDIES FOR A STARTER KIT

The following list contains some of the most frequently used homeopathic medicines for menopausal complaints, as well as a range of other conditions such as accidents, injuries, stomach disorders, and joint problems. Because of the multifaceted nature of homeopathic medicines, you will find that a remedy such as

Arsenicum album may be used for anxiety, food poisoning, sore throats, coughs, flu, or cystitis, provided the symptoms of the remedy match those of the patient. You will therefore find that your basic range of remedies, although initially chosen to help with menopausal problems, will be appropriate for treating a range of additional problems.

If you are interested in using your remedies in a broader context, you will need a general guide to homeopathic prescribing for acute conditions or a number of individual books that deal with specific conditions, such as children's ailments, accidents and sports injuries, or women's health. A list of appropriate guides is given in the further reading section.

The suggested remedies for your starter kit should include:

Aconite	Ignatia
Arnica	Lachesis
Arsenicum album	Natrum mur.
Belladonna	Nux vomica
Calc. carb.	Pulsatilla
Gelsemium	Sepia

Once you have this basic kit, the following will be useful additions:

Anacardium	Lycopodium
Arg. nit.	Phosphorus
Bryonia	Rhus tox.
Causticum	Staphysagria
Cimicifuga	Sulphur
Kali. carb.	

It is important to remember that this is by no means an exhaustive list, and that there are many important homeopathic medicines that I have not mentioned. However, if you combine these two remedy selections, you should have a good working kit that will meet most eventualities.

In addition, it is helpful to have the following items in your basic kit:

Calendula or Hypercal™ cream
Calendula or Hypercal™ tincture (to be diluted)

Both of these can be applied as local preparations to the skin where soreness, inflammation, or itching have occurred.

FINDING OUT MORE ABOUT HOMEOPATHIC SELF-HELP

If you enjoy using this book, and feel you would like to expand your knowledge of homeopathy, you would benefit from attending one of the many homeopathic self-help courses that are regularly run throughout the country. Most of these will be taught by professional homeopaths, who can guide you through the practical issues connected with self-help prescribing, as well as explaining the basic principles of homeopathic philosophy. Attending a class of this kind can be great fun, as well as giving you an important opportunity to raise questions or queries in connection with your own experience of homeopathic prescribing. They are also excellent places for building confidence in using self-help measures, since shared positive experiences are very exciting, empowering, and exhilarating.

If you would like to find out more about self-help classes in your area, contact your local library or adult education department at your local university or college for further information. Inquire if there is a homeopathic college or training center near you, since they are often very helpful in giving information about beginners' courses in homeopathy.

CONDITIONS THAT REQUIRE PROFESSIONAL HELP

The suggestion is made at certain points in this book that you need to seek professional homeopathic help. This is because certain conditions or stages of ill health should not be handled by the layperson or newcomer to homeopathic prescribing. These illnesses can be described as *chronic*. Conditions that fall into the chronic category include rheumatoid arthritis, asthma, hay fever, depression, migraines, stomach ulcers, irritable bowel syndrome, and eczema. All these conditions have in common a tendency to flare up repeatedly, often increasing gradually in severity, with no tendency for the condition to resolve itself decisively.

Acute conditions, on the other hand, have a limited duration and resolve themselves decisively, provided the body is given the best conditions in which to do so. Good examples of acute conditions include the common cold, flu, food poisoning, and digestive upsets from an unusual amount of overindulgence. These are the ideal conditions with which to build up confidence in self-prescribing, since positive reactions are often rapid and impressive.

However, there are also problems that fall in an intermediate category, being neither clear-cut acute nor chronic conditions. These include illnesses that happen infrequently, at a very low level, or in association with a general process, such as vaginal irritation after menopause. A selection of these problems will be found in this book, as well as some conditions that would normally fall into the chronic category, such as varicose veins, depression, anxiety, and arthritis. Although the latter conditions are best treated by a professional for the most positive outcome in the long term, if symptoms are mild or intermittent, a great deal may be gained by making general positive changes in lifestyle, and occasional homeopathic self-prescribing. However, always remember that homeopathic medicines are not intended to be taken over an extended period but should be used only infrequently. If you find you need to take them constantly to sustain an improvement, it is best to consult a homeopathic practitioner.

For many of us, the degree of short-term relief we experience as a result of making these changes may be the impetus that leads us to explore more holistic approaches to healing and health care. As always, if you feel confused or out of your depth when using homeopathic self-help techniques, always seek professional advice rather than soldiering on alone.

FINDING A HOMEOPATHIC PRACTITIONER

Although registers can be helpful in providing reassurance that a homeopath has recognized qualifications, the best way of finding a practitioner is often by word of mouth. If a family member, friend, or colleague has been treated by a responsible, professional, and empathetic homeopath, it is worth making further inquiries. Most homeopaths or receptionists will be happy to give details of costs of treatment over the telephone as well as answering any other practical inquiries that may arise. Personal recommendation is also an excellent way of overcoming the fact that there are capable and well-respected practitioners who may have trained before the college system was set up or the registration process began.

If you do not have access to a personal recommendation, you may wish to consult the International Foundation for Homeopathy or the National Center for Homeopathy (see the Resources section, p. 220). Both organizations can provide additional information about the practice of homeopathy in the United States.

TAKING CONVENTIONAL MEDICATION AND HOMEOPATHIC MEDICINES

Homeopathic medicines work on a level totally different from that of conventional drugs. Because of their infinitesimal degree of dilution, they are not working in a chemically detectable way in the tissues of our bodies. As a result, there is little chance of their having an adverse reaction with orthodox drugs, in the obvious sense that toxic chemicals might react badly when mixed together.

However, there are more subtle arguments that suggest that drugs that have a powerful effect on our immune systems, such as antibiotics, may disrupt the effective action of homeopathic medicines. This is thought to be especially the case with steroid formulations. Steroids have a spectacular ability to suppress symptoms, and, as a result, have a formidable immunosuppressive action on our bodies. Treating patients who are on such powerful medication with homeopathic medicines can be very difficult, since it is often an uphill struggle to work out which symptoms belong to the original complaint and which are side effects of the conventional medication.

Nevertheless, homeopaths are often faced with the reality of treating patients who are taking orthodox drugs. In this situation, it is often necessary to attempt homeopathic treatment alongside conventional therapy, especially if patients are taking drugs that cannot be withdrawn rapidly. Once improvement occurs, it may become possible to withdraw conventional medication slowly and responsibly, ideally with the consent and supervision of the physician who prescribed the orthodox treatment.

If you are a beginner in homeopathic self-prescribing, it is best to wait until you have finished a short course of previously prescribed orthodox medication (such as antibiotics) before you begin. On the other hand, if you are taking conventional drugs on a permanent basis, you have little to lose by trying a strongly indicated homeopathic remedy. If you feel you respond well to your selected remedy and want to cut down your orthodox medication, do not act rashly. It must be stressed that drugs such as steroids, antidepressants, and high or regular doses of tranquilizers should never be withdrawn abruptly or without medical supervision. Always seek professional advice if you are in any doubt about conventional or homeopathic medication.

21

3

~

Emotional Reactions
to Menopause

Although some of us pass through menopause with very little disruption, others may suffer confusing emotional reactions to the physical changes that are occurring in our bodies. For those who experience these transient problems, homeopathy can play an extremely positive role by supporting us through the turbulence of mood swings and emotional imbalances. By opting for this approach, we avoid the undesirable side effects, such as drowsiness or dependency, of some conventional medical treatments.

It is as appropriate to seek homeopathic help for emotional problems as it is for physical disorders, since homeopaths place great emphasis on emotional well-being as the foundation of good health. Many patients arrive at a practitioner's office expecting to talk exclusively about their physical symptoms. As the consultation progresses, they are often surprised to discover that their homeopath is as interested in their emotional well-being (or imbalance) as in their stomach disorder or their joint pains. This information is invaluable, since the homeopath can use it as a yardstick to determine how well a patient is progressing towards cure once treatment has begun. In other words, there must be a marked improvement right across the board, with emotional imbalances improving in proportion to the relief of physical problems, before well-established progress is made.

If you suffer from mild or infrequent problems with any of the

22

conditions discussed in this chapter, you may find that homeopathic self-prescribing and practical self-help measures may be all
you need to regain your equilibrium. However, if you have experienced any of these problems for a long time or if your symptoms
are severe, you should seek help from a trained homeopathic
practitioner to ensure the best possible outcome.

In this chapter you will find a survey of emotional conditions,
giving positive advice from a homeopathic and general self-help
perspective. As always, consult the practical information given in
chapter 2. By being familiar with the instructions given in this section, you are most likely to experience a positive result.

ANXIETY

Although we can feel anxious at any age, the years immediately
before and after menopause are a time when our anxiety levels
can be especially high. Feeling panicky, tense, or frightened are
common symptoms that may accompany hot flashes or night
sweats. In some instances, we may find that we experience a wave
of foreboding or uneasiness before a hot flash begins, almost as a
form of early warning signal.

The degree of anxiety that we experience can vary enormously
from vague feelings of uneasiness to outright panic. Although the
variation is great, the following can be identified as common
symptoms of anxiety:

• light-headedness or dizziness;
• palpitations or rapid pulse;
• nausea;
• weak, trembly limbs;
• dry mouth;
• rapid, shallow breathing;
• diarrhea;

- alternating heat and chills;
- a feeling of wanting to escape or run away;
- feeling frightened or panicked for no obvious reason.

Although these symptoms can be immensely distressing, we can benefit greatly from practical self-help measures, which can reduce the frequency and severity of attacks.

Homeopathic Help

If you feel occasionally anxious under pressure or uneasy for no obvious reason, one of the homeopathic remedies shown in the following table may help a great deal in calming you down. It is a good idea to take your remedy as soon as you feel tense or before an event that you know is going to be a source of stress or anxiety. Take your remedy only when you feel anxious; once an improvement takes place, this is a sign that your body can now cope on its own and no further stimulation is needed from a homeopathic medicine, unless and until your symptoms return.

If you need to repeat your selected remedy frequently to maintain an improvement or if a well-selected homeopathic medicine does not result in improvement, you should seek professional help. This does not mean that homeopathy cannot help you, merely that you need a more experienced perspective on your symptoms as a whole.

Practical Self-Help

BREATHING

If you feel anxious, observe how you are breathing. Most of us breathe rapidly and shallowly from our upper chests when feeling threatened, without realizing that this makes the situation worse. By breathing in this way, we adversely affect the ratio of oxygen and carbon dioxide in our bodies, with the result that we feel even more tense and jittery and breathe even faster. We can do a great deal to calm ourselves by learning how to breathe in a way that induces relaxation and clarity of thought. We can achieve this by learning a simple technique called diaphragmatic breathing and using it whenever we feel stressed, anxious, or panicked.

You can practice this invaluable self-help measure by resting your hand lightly on your navel as you sit in a straight-backed chair. Relax and breathe out completely as you become aware of any areas of tension in your body. When you breathe in, feel the air filling your upper chest, slowly inflating your lungs until your hand is pushed gently upward and outward. Pause for a second, then slowly exhale from the base of the lungs, expelling air finally from the upper chest. As you do this, your hand should sink back down again. If you find this difficult at first, it may help to press down gently as you begin to exhale. This should quickly become unnecessary as you become familiar with the feeling of breathing from your abdomen rather than your upper chest. Breathe easily, evenly, and slowly, never forcing the process but allowing it to happen at its own pace. If you feel light-headed or dizzy, return to normal breathing patterns for a while until you feel more settled. Once you have mastered this technique, you can use it any time you feel tension or anxiety developing.

RELAXATION

Exploring relaxation, visualization, or meditation techniques can also be an excellent way of diffusing stress or anxiety. You might want to start by using one of the many audiocassettes available, which will talk you through a guided relaxation exercise. If you prefer a more personal approach, a good yoga teacher should provide an extended relaxation session at the end of each class.

Become aware of the parts of your body that tighten up when you become anxious or tense. Common areas affected by muscular tension include the jaw, the muscles at either side of the neck, and

Typical Features	*General Symptoms*
Sudden descending terror with fear of death	Panic attacks come on rapidly with little or no warning. Physically and mentally restless with conviction that death is near. Skin is flushed and dry, or may alternate between heat and chill. Feels worse if approached.
Anxiety with digestive upsets, e.g., nausea, vomiting, or diarrhea	Anxious and fearful feelings accompany a threat to routine or feeling in control. Always worried about untidiness, germs, or ill health. Fears are much worse at night and in the dark when no one else is around. Waves of burning heat alternate with icy chills.
Anxiety with severe digestive problems, e.g., rumbling and gurgling	Constantly driven by nervousness, and cannot do things fast enough to keep up. Very nervous and fearful before any event that is likely to be demanding. Fears being closed in, heights, or crowds. Craves sugar, which makes everything worse.
Anticipatory anxiety about speaking in public	Although tense and nervous before public speaking, all goes well when it happens. Outwardly seems confident and in command, but inwardly very nervous. Waist and abdomen swell when nervous, so that a tight waistband must be loosened.
Withdrawn, silent, and preoccupied with anxiety	Although internally agitated, appears apathetic and weary. Lacks interest in conversation and surroundings. Severe, painless diarrhea when tense. Anxiety may build slowly with progressive trembling of hands.
Anxious and short-tempered from overuse of coffee and alcohol	High strung, nervous, and tense when feeling overworked and overburdened. Needs coffee to keep going, alcohol to relax, and frequent painkillers for headaches. Flies off the handle when stress gets too much. Unrelaxed and wakeful at night, with palpitations.

Emotional Reactions to Menopause

Better for	Worse from	Remedy
Fresh air Sweating Moderate temperatures	Shock or fright Exposure to cold, sharp winds Drinking wine Becoming overheated At night	Aconite
Warmth Sips of warm drinks Sweating	Cold Being alone At night Alcohol	Arsenicum album
Cool, fresh air Light clothes Walking in the open air	Warmth Stuffy rooms Stress of any kind On waking Sugar	Argentum nit.
Moderate temperatures Warm food and drinks Loosening clothing Being occupied Exercise in the open air	Hot, stuffy rooms Being chilled Emotional stress	Lycopodium
Fresh air Sweating Gentle exercise	Overheating Chills Brooding	Gelsemium
Warmth A sound sleep Being left alone As the day goes on	Being cold or chilled Coffee Alcohol In the morning Noise Interrupted sleep	Nux vomica

the shoulders, arms, and hands. Next time you feel anxious, take a moment to observe how you are holding yourself. There is every likelihood that your jaw is tight and clenched, your shoulders are raised up toward your ears, and your fingers may be held in a fist. Breathe out slowly and fully, and consciously let your jaw relax. As a result, your shoulders should sink down away from your ears, and the muscles in your arms and hands will relax. If you combine this awareness with the breathing exercise outlined above, you will have a simple but effective way of relaxing your mind and body that can be used at any time you feel stressed.

EXERCISE

Be aware of the reaction called the "fight or flight response" and the value of physical exercise in dealing with it. When we feel stressed or threatened, the body responds by preparing itself for physical effort. As a result, the heart beats faster, more blood is pumped to the muscles, and blood pressure rises. While this response may be perfectly appropriate if we need to sprint away from a physically threatening situation, reacting this way when faced with financial or domestic worries can lead to a variety of stress-related health problems. These may include high blood pressure, anxiety, digestive disorders such as indigestion and nausea, and chronic headaches and migraines. On the other hand, if we increase our physical activity through regular exercise, we can channel these stress-induced reactions in a more appropriate way, thus reducing our risk of anxiety and related health problems.

DIET

A number of foods can aggravate feelings of stress and anxiety. These include caffeine (which may aggravate palpitations and sleep problems), alcohol, sugary cakes, drinks, and cookies, and chocolate. Switch to soothing herbal drinks such as camomile tea and eat plenty of whole foods and regular helpings of fresh fruit, raw or lightly cooked vegetables, and salads. If you find it difficult to give up carbonated drinks, switch to carbonated water with a dash of lemon or choose some of the new varieties of carbonated soft drinks with fruit juices and no added sugar or artificial sweeteners such as aspartame or saccharine.

Consider supplementing your diet with vitamins from the B complex, which help maintain the health of our nervous systems. It is best to use a B complex formulation, rather than a single B vitamin in high dosage. This is because there is a risk of toxic side effects from large doses of vitamin B_6, and because the B vitamins seem to work most effectively when given in complex formulation.

AROMATHERAPY
Use soothing and relaxing essential oils in a relaxing bath before a stressful event or whenever you feel tension is building. A few drops of any of the following may be helpful: neroli, camomile, sandalwood, or rose. These oils are extremely concentrated, and very small quantities are needed to produce the desired effect.

"EMPTY NEST" SYNDROME

Although menopause can be a potentially very exciting time when we have a chance to expand our horizons, it can also result in our feeling vulnerable and bereft. This can be particularly marked if menopause swiftly follows or coincides with our children becoming independent and leaving home.

While many of us come to relish the freedom that this brings, most of us go through a transitory phase of conflicting emotions before the positive side of the situation becomes apparent. The imbalance is often made worse by the emotional tugs of war and battles of will that ensue between parents and teenagers. These conflicts usually precede our children's final assertion of independence by making a home of their own.

Some of us may respond to this situation by wanting to return to the past, while others may feel a strong urge to have a baby in an attempt to start all over again. These feelings may often be further complicated by the demands that are made by elderly parents as they face the anxieties of getting older. Where these demands amount to dependency, the role reversal can be very painful, and many of us may feel overwhelmed by the weight of responsibility.

Common symptoms of "empty nest" syndrome are:

- low libido and vitality;
- abrupt mood swings and weepiness for no obvious reason;
- poor quality or disrupted sleep pattern;
- a general feeling of depression, which may be especially marked on waking;
- indifference or lack of motivation;
- inability to concentrate;
- general aches and pains or muscular tension;
- comfort eating, with resultant weight gain, or, in contrast, a complete lack of interest in food.

Homeopathic Help

Although no form of medication can take problems or excessive responsibilities away, there is a great deal that sound homeopathic prescribing can do to support us through traumatic times. Although the demands will still be there, such help will give us greater resilience and so enable us to cope better. An appropriately prescribed homeopathic medicine gives our physical and emotional energy levels a much-needed boost, and we often find that problems that seemed insoluble now appear less threatening because our perspective has changed. Once we have a calmer and more objective view of the problem, we have a much better chance of working it out.

If you feel infrequent or mild episodes of distress at the prospect of your children leaving home, an occasional dose of the most appropriate homeopathic medicine selected from the table below may help you overcome the temporary crisis. However, if you are concerned about the severity or long-term nature of your symptoms or you feel that they are radically altering the quality of your life in an adverse way, it is essential to seek professional advice.

Practical Self-Help

SELF-DEVELOPMENT

Consider taking up interests that you may have neglected while your children were growing up or developing new skills that are attractive to you. By concentrating on exploring new areas of interest, this phase of your life can be transformed into an exciting and challenging new start. Adult education courses can provide the opportunity to update existing qualifications or open up fresh areas of interest. Attending classes of this kind can also give us the added bonus of putting us in touch with a new circle of friends. As a result, we are likely to find that we are given a new lease of life at a time when we least expected it.

Take advantage of your new-found freedom by doing some of the traveling you may have put off while you were responsible for a young family.

COMMUNICATION

Talk to your partner about how he feels now that your children are ready to leave home. You may be surprised to find that he is going through similar emotions as yourself but may not be inclined to initiate talking it through. Sadly, many men still suffer the legacy of needing to keep a "stiff upper lip" in the face of emotional strain or bereavement. As a result, they may interpret open emotional responses such as tearfulness as a sign of weakness

Typical Features	*General Symptoms*
Very weepy with little or no control over bouts of crying	Has bouts of sadness and distress that cannot be resolved. Moods are changeable; sometimes laughs one moment and cries the next. Tense and anxious when emotionally upset. Sighs or yawns constantly, and may have spasmodic bouts of hiccups when upset.
Suppressed anger with sadness	Inwardly tense and angry at children for leaving, but remains sweet and calm on the surface. Anger comes to the surface if pushed to the emotional limit. Explosive temper, causing trembling and shaking through whole body.
Weepy, irritable, and apathetic toward sexual partner	Unhappy and depressed and feels that family demands are too much. Low-spirited and tends to snap at the slightest provocation. Displays of affection and sexual activity make things worse.
Weepy and sad with a need for sympathy and affection	Moods change rapidly from anxiety and irritability to sadness. Frequently bursts into tears, which give relief. Feels better when in sympathetic company.
Irritable and stressed from becoming "burned out" at work	Overcommitment to work has become a substitute for family life. Hard to relax at night, which often leads to chronic insomnia. May be dependent on sleeping pills, alcohol, or painkillers in order to cope.
Constant, underlying general anxiety that surfaces when upset	Insecure, anxious, and in need of reassurance when faced with the trauma of children leaving home. Sensitive to others' moods and to general atmospheres. Needs to be calmed down when distressed. Can alternate rapidly between enthusiasm and boredom.

Emotional Reactions to Menopause

Better for	Worse from	Remedy
Warmth Distraction Eating	Cold Tobacco, alcohol, or coffee Sensory stimulation	Ignatia
After eating Resting Sleep	Emotional strain Early morning Light touch Tobacco	Staphysagria
Sleep Vigorous, aerobic exercise Fresh air Warmth	Emotional strain Sitting and brooding Before a period	Sepia
Cool food and drinks Cool, fresh air Gentle exercise Sympathy and attention Having a good cry	Stuffy, overheated rooms In the evening Becoming chilled Being alone Lying in bed	Pulsatilla
Warmth Sound sleep Being left in peace By the evening	Stress Coffee Being disturbed Cold, drafty surroundings In the morning	Nux vomica

Reassurance
Massage and physical
    affection
Warmth
Good quality sleep
	Overexcitement or
	    -stimulation
	Crowds
	In the evenings
	Darkness
	Being alone
		Phosphorus

or undesirable vulnerability. By communicating openly with your partner about your own confusion, fear, sadness, anger, or ambivalence about the maturing of your children, you may be surprised at the positive outcome. This communication may bring you much closer together as you experience a shared understanding of the situation.

DIET

This is a time when you need to ensure that you are not neglecting your diet and that you are gaining maximum benefit and support from a nutritious eating plan. Avoid food and drinks that have a reputation for aggravating mood swings: these include alcohol, very sugary drinks and foods, strong coffee, prepared foods, and chocolate. If you feel your diet has suffered over the recent months, you could consider supplementing with vitamin B complex and vitamin C to give you a temporary boost.

EXERCISE

Take up regular physical exercise. This may be one of your new interests such as joining a tennis or squash club or attending a gym or low-impact aerobics class. When we are physically fitter we begin to feel more energized, confident, and ready to face the future.

Counseling

If your symptoms are becoming a long-term problem and do not respond to self-help measures, you may benefit a great deal from counseling. Very often, talking about our feelings to a therapist who is free from emotional involvement in our problems can lead to an immense sense of relief. It may also enable us to see our situation from a different, more balanced perspective.

DEPRESSION

Depression may strike us at any time, but menopause is a phase of life when we may be prone to develop feelings of sadness or depression. These feelings may be occasional or frequent, transient or long-lasting. They are due to the fluctuations in hormone levels that occur at this time, and those of us who suffered symptoms of premenstrual syndrome (PMS) or postnatal depression in the past may be more at risk.

The symptoms of depression can vary greatly in severity and in their general nature. Common symptoms include:

- an all-pervading sense of hopelessness, sadness, or apathy that can descend without warning or obvious reason;
- extreme or rapidly alternating mood swings;
- disturbed, unrefreshing, or poor-quality sleep, with anxiety or sadness on waking;
- lack of interest in sex;
- disrupted eating patterns with tendency for comfort eating or total lack of interest in food;
- digestive problems including nausea, heartburn, indigestion, or irritable bowel syndrome;
- palpitations, anxiety, or rapid breathing from the upper chest;
- dizziness, light-headedness, or lack of concentration.

Homeopathic Help

It is important to differentiate between transient depression, which lifts as a result of self-help measures, and a more long-term tendency to a depressive state. For the former, there is a great deal that can be done with occasional homeopathic prescribing and the use of supportive practical self-help. If you find that your symptoms are interfering with your day-to-day life, if things are getting

Typical Features	*General Symptoms*
Withdrawn and depressed with a need to be alone	Inclined to bottle up emotions and take things to heart. Feels much worse for crying in front of people, especially if they offer sympathy. Depression may follow a long-term emotional strain or bereavement where feelings have been repressed.
Lacks motivation and interest in anything	Depression is bleak but relieved by vigorous exercise. May be irritable and aggressive with family or totally apathetic toward them. Although feeling antisocial, fears being alone. Feels out of control and unable to cope. A total lack of interest in sex when depressed.
Black, gloomy depression alternates with being totally high strung	Extremely restless when depressed, with strong fear of death or insanity. Feels out of control and frantic. Moods alternate rapidly between total misery, marked anxiety, and euphoria. Feels better emotionally when physical symptoms emerge.
Restless depression with acute anxiety about health	Physically and mentally driven, with fear of losing control. Depression may develop because of an inability to reach own high standards. Self-critical and intolerant of others, with a terror of failure. Chilly and nauseated, with insomnia when depressed.
Depression on waking that improves as the day goes on	Rapid changes of mood, with a tendency to be irritable, chatty, cutting, aggressive, jealous, or anxious. Subject to a flow of creative ideas at night, and a dislike of falling asleep. Full of ideas, but finds it difficult to carry them through.
Hopeless depression that descends in bed at night	Extremely restless and wakeful during the night. Worries and feels despondent about work and family commitments, and anxious about the future. Becomes tearful for no obvious reason, and feels despairing about everything. Physical problems such as joint pains or itchy skin contribute to restlessness and wakefulness.

Emotional Reactions to Menopause

Better for	Worse from	Remedy
Privacy Cool surroundings Skipping meals Gentle exercise	Attention and sympathy After weeping Heat or direct sunlight Physical effort Displays of affection	Natrum mur.

A sound sleep
Resting in a warm bed
Fresh air
Exercise such as brisk
  walking or running in
  the fresh air
Eating regularly
	Sitting still
	Skipping meals
	Meeting emotional needs
	  of family
		Sepia

Warmth Fresh air Eating Walking	Damp and cold After resting Before a period Night	Cimicifuga
Warmth Being propped-up in bed Company Warm drinks or food Moving about	At night Cold in any form Being alone Alcohol	Arsenicum album
Cool, fresh air Loose clothing Onset of a period Movement Cool drinks	Warm, stuffy rooms Feeling constricted Before a period Extreme changes of temperature	Lachesis
Warmth Warm bathing Continued movement Wrapping up snugly	Cold and damp Resting Overexertion At night	Rhus tox.

worse, if you need to repeat your selected homeopathic medicine on a long-term basis to gain relief, or if you have a history of long-term depression and are taking orthodox medication, it is important that you seek help from a trained practitioner. This also applies if you have suffered from long-term anxiety in the past. Well-established depression and anxiety constitute a chronic emotional condition, which it is not appropriate to handle by self-prescribing. An experienced homeopathic practitioner, on the other hand, will treat the whole person on emotional, mental, and physical levels and is trained to prescribe accordingly.

Practical Self-Help

COMMUNICATION

If you feel low, talk it over with a close friend, family member, or your partner. Don't fall into the trap of thinking that it is best to keep our feelings to ourselves; we may store up problems for the future if our feelings are unacknowledged. If you prefer not to talk over your troubles with someone who is close to you, consider seeing a counselor who will be able to take a more objective stance when listening to your problems.

RELAXATION

Treat yourself with as much kindness as you would give to a close friend if she or he were feeling unhappy. When we feel down, it is very tempting to be much more critical of ourselves than we would ever dream of being with anyone else. Make time for yourself, and do things that you enjoy. This may be as simple as taking a long walk each day, listening to a favorite piece of music, or reading a book.

AROMATHERAPY

Use aromatherapy as a way of uplifting your spirits. Add a few drops to your bath water, in a carrier oil massaged into your skin, or burned on a warm lightbulb ring. Oils to consider include neroli, jasmine, geranium, rose, or ylang-ylang.

DIET

Be aware that certain foods can help or hinder us when we are feeling depressed. The helpful foods include those that give us as broad a range of essential nutrients as possible, such as whole grains, fresh fruit, vegetables, fish, pulses, beans, poultry, and small quantities of dairy foods. Those to avoid include alcohol, sugary foods and drinks, coffee, strong tea, chocolate, and junk foods such as prepared foods containing artificial flavorings, colorings, and preservatives, potato chips and other salty snacks, and convenience foods containing a high proportion of refined sugar, flour and/or fat.

Consider taking a B complex vitamin supplement to support your nervous system or a good quality multivitamin if you feel your eating patterns have become irregular since feeling depressed.

EXERCISE

If you are feeling depressed, there is a tremendous amount to be gained from becoming physically active. Regular, rhythmic exercise stimulates our bodies to secrete endorphins, which are chemicals that resemble natural antidepressants. These are responsible for the "high" that many of us may have experienced after running, cycling, or an aerobics class. When we exercise our hearts and lungs in this way, our bodies make maximum use of the oxygen we take in. This is a vital detoxifying process, which also contributes to a feeling of vitality, alertness, and overall well-being.

If we exercise regularly, we often experience the added bonus of feeling more positive about our bodies and experiencing increased overall physical stamina and condition. This can provide us with a powerful and welcome confidence boost when our self-esteem may be low.

Remember that you should not be overambitious to start with: begin by taking a regular, brisk walk each day. As this becomes an established part of your routine, you can consider other forms of exercise that appeal to you. Don't limit yourself, but consider the full range of possibilities. Opt for something enjoyable and fun that expands your social circle as well. If you choose in this way, you are most likely to stick to whatever you have decided to do.

4

~

General Problems

In this chapter we will look at a range of general conditions that we are likely to experience in the premenopausal or post-menopausal years. Although there may be a slight overlap with the problems outlined in chapter 5, the conditions described in this section are generally more diffused and less likely to affect a specific organ or system of our bodies in isolation.

As a rule, the more a problem affects our overall experience of health, the more holistic our approach to healing needs to be. In other words, we need to take a positive stance about changes in our general lifestyle as well as to consider self-help support from homeopathic prescribing. By doing so, we begin to discover that a homeopathic perspective of healing is not restricted to eradicating individual symptoms, but is much more concerned with elevating our sense of well-being and general health.

In this chapter you will find a survey of general problems that may limit our sense of vitality and zest for life. Because of the need for a holistic approach, positive advice is given from both a homeopathic and general self-help perspective. As always, consult the practical information given in chapter 2. If you are familiar with the instructions given in this section, you are most likely to experience a positive outcome.

GENERAL FATIGUE AND LOW ENERGY LEVELS

Although exhaustion can hit us at any time in our lives, there are specific life events that are especially associated with erratic or reduced energy levels. These include puberty, pregnancy, the initial months following childbirth, and menopause. Each of these profound phases of development involves a radical shift in hormonal levels as well as the need to come to terms with new challenges, responsibilities, and relationships.

Although it is in the nature of change to be stimulating and exciting, it can also be confusing, alarming, and exhausting if we do not have the support to help us make the most of it. This can be especially true of the premenopausal years, which involve physical and emotional changes that at times can leave us feeling wrung out. On the other hand, there is an enormous amount we can do to support ourselves through these years by making simple changes that will boost our energy levels so that we can cope with the challenges presented to us as they arise.

Homeopathic Help

Because homeopathic medicines work by stimulating our energy levels and activating the self-healing potential that we all possess, successful homeopathic prescribing should always result in enhanced vitality and well-being on physical, emotional, and mental levels. This far-reaching and ambitious goal is most likely to be attained by receiving professional help from a trained practitioner, who will be working at a "constitutional" level, attempting to restore your system as a whole to its optimum state of harmony and balance.

However, if you are subject to mild or short-lived feelings of fatigue, you can achieve a great deal with basic self-help measures and a short-term prescription of an appropriate homeopathic remedy. Remember that homeopathic remedies are not designed to be taken over a long period. If you find you need to take your remedy frequently to maintain an improvement, you should seek professional advice. This does not mean that homeopathy is not suitable for you, but that you may need a different dosage or remedy to deal with the root of your problem.

Practical Self-Help

EXERCISE

Although you may not be keen on the idea when you feel lethargic, regular exercise is one of your most important allies in the fight against flagging energy levels. Regular, enjoyable, rhythmic exercise not only diffuses stress and anxiety levels but also stimulates endorphin production. Remember from chapter 3 that endorphins are natural antidepressants that give pleasurable or pain-relieving sensations and the uplift that many of us have experienced after aerobic exercise.

It is essential that you choose an activity that you find exhilarating, challenging, and enjoyable so that you don't become bored very quickly. Possible options are swimming, cycling, tennis, volleyball, walking, or low-impact aerobics. Combine activities that get your lungs and heart working with stretching exercises that encourage flexibility, increased muscular strength, and stamina. Attending a yoga class is an excellent way of combining effective stretching exercises with relaxation and breathing techniques.

DIET

Be aware of foods and drinks that boost your energy level and those that drain it. Foods that enhance vitality include whole grains, fresh fruit and vegetables, pulses (beans, peas, and lentils), and fish and poultry in moderation. Energy-reducing foods include sweetened drinks, chocolate, cakes, cookies, strong coffee or tea, alcohol, convenience foods, red meat, and high-fat foods such as dairy products.

Avoid falling into the trap of assuming that lots of sugary foods

Typical Features	**General Symptoms**
Easily exhausted with a tendency to gain weight easily	Chilly but perspires quickly after the least physical effort. Feels worse during or after exercise. Body functions sluggishly, leading to slow metabolism, poor circulation, and constipation.
Exhaustion that is improved by vigorous exercise	Depressed, apathetic, and unsociable with fatigue. Everything feels heavy and drooping. Aggressive toward or lacks interest in partner. Low libido. Headaches and nausea, with extreme tiredness from low blood-sugar levels.
Anxious and physically restless with tiredness	Cannot rest in one place although exhausted. Has to plan and organize constantly to feel in control. Once control slips, anxiety sets in. Nausea and diarrhea with extreme tiredness. Physical discomfort if cold.
Periodic tiredness each afternoon, lasting until evening	Tired and anxious with digestive problems that are worse before an event. Stomach rumbles, gurgles, and feels bloated. Craves sugar and sweet things to keep going.
Irritable and excitable from excess physical and mental stress	Exhausted after "burning the candle at both ends." Relies on stimulants, painkillers, and alcohol to keep the pace. As a result, constipation, headaches, indigestion, and insomnia are a persistent problem.
Slow-developing tiredness with headaches or dizziness	Weariness with heavy limbs and aching muscles. The slightest job requires enormous effort because of lack of energy. Shivery and chilly with tiredness. Headache with tight sensation in forehead above the eyes.
Weary and weepy with a strong need for consolation	Chilly, dizzy, and faint, especially in stuffy, airless atmospheres. Although tired at night, cannot get into a deep, refreshing sleep. Shifting, changeable aches and pains.

Better for	Worse from	Remedy
Resting Moderate warmth Constipation	Exposure to cold and damp Physical exercise Standing Before or during a period Being observed	Calc. carb.
Aerobic exercise Fresh air Being warm in bed Eating Sleep	Sitting still Before a period Emotional demands Skipping meals	Sepia
Warm rooms Hot water bottle Sitting propped up in bed Warm drinks	Chilly rooms Cold drinks Alcohol At night Being alone	Arsenicum album
Fresh air Warm drinks Moderate warmth Being occupied Gentle exercise Loosening clothing	Emotional strain or stress Pressure Stuffy rooms Tight clothing On waking In the afternoon	Lycopodium
Sleep Warmth Being left in peace Lying down As the day goes on	Alcohol Coffee After eating Mental strain Broken sleep On waking	Nux vomica
Fresh air Gentle, continued movement Perspiring Passing urine	Becoming overheated Damp conditions Cold drafts	Gelsemium
Fresh, open air Cool surroundings Cool drinks Gentle exercise Sympathy Having a good cry	Warmth At night Being still Heavy clothes or bed covers Rich, fatty foods	Pulsatilla

and drinks provide extra energy: unfortunately the reverse is true. Each time we take sugar in the form of cakes, cookies, chocolate bars or soft drinks, our blood sugar levels rise dramatically, giving an initial boost. Our bodies respond by secreting insulin to bring down the level of sugar in the blood, resulting in a loss of energy and poor concentration. A common response to this light-headed or lethargic feeling is to reach for another sugar boost. This leads to a perpetual cycle of sugar consumption, in which we need increasingly large sugar fixes to keep going.

BREATHING

Concentrate on breathing techniques that enable you to make maximum use of the oxygen that you breathe in. Always ensure that you breathe out fully before breathing in, so that you make full use of your lung capacity. If you are feeling anxious, be aware that your breathing rate may be more rapid and shallow than normal, resulting in an imbalance in levels of carbon dioxide and oxygen in your body. By regulating your breathing pattern, making it deeper and slower, you will feel calmer, clear-headed, and more in control. If you are interested in learning more about breathing techniques, consider attending a yoga class or take a look at the increasing number of audiocassettes on the market that guide you through a relaxation or meditation session.

AROMATHERAPY

Use aromatherapy oils creatively, adding a few drops to your bathwater, massaging them into your skin in a carrier-oil base, or burning a few drops on a lightbulb ring to scent your room. Essential oils that have an invigorating and stimulating effect include: rosemary, peppermint, coriander, eucalyptus, and citrus essences.

SKIN CARE

Dry skin brushing is an excellent way of stimulating the lymph system and encouraging increased elimination of toxic waste from the skin. Smooth functioning of our lymphatic system helps to protect us against recurrent infections and disease, as well as guarding against chronic lethargy and tiredness. Always brush your skin with a natural bristle brush or a dry hemp glove, using firm but not harsh strokes. Use sweeping movements, moving up the legs and arms and down the torso. Avoid brushing any areas with irritated, sensitive, or broken skin.

SLEEP
Refreshing sleep is a basic foundation of sustained energy levels and a general sense of well-being. If you feel a poor sleep pattern is your problem, follow the advice given in the following section.

INSOMNIA AND DISTURBED SLEEP PATTERN

Many women who had no sleep problems in their youth are surprised and anxious to find that they experience a poor or disturbed sleep pattern as they approach menopause. The degree of disturbance can vary enormously, from difficulties in falling asleep to an interrupted rest where we wake up every hour or two. Even if broken sleep is not a problem, the quality or depth of it may be adversely affected, leaving us feeling unrefreshed on waking.

Homeopathic Help

Well-prescribed homeopathic medicines can be immensely helpful in easing sleep problems without the side effects, such as drowsiness or addiction, of narcotic drugs. As always, the selected remedy must fit individual symptoms very closely for it to be effective. If you find that you need to take a homeopathic medicine on a long-term basis to maintain an improvement, it is important that you seek professional help from a homeopathic practitioner, who will be able to prescribe in a more precise way,

Typical Features	**General Symptoms**
Wakes around 1:00 to 3:00 A.M. feeling very anxious	Physically and mentally restless in bed. Gets up to walk around or make a cup of tea. Feels calm through the day, but becomes increasingly anxious as the night goes on.
Fitful sleep with dependence on sedatives to relax	Difficult to "switch off" from domestic worries or stresses at work. Uses caffeine to keep alert through the day, causing wakefulness at night. Irritable, headachy and constipated as a result of overstressful lifestyle.
Sensations of falling or suffocation on falling asleep	Dreads going to bed because of feelings associated with falling asleep or waking. Holds breath while falling asleep, and wakes suddenly with a jerk or jolting sensation. Confused, headachy, and unrefreshed on waking. Hot flashes or night sweats may prevent or disturb sleep.
Insomnia with severe anxiety and fear	Very drowsy during the day but wide awake at night. May wake from sleep after nightmares or disturbing dreams. Sleep problems may follow a frightening experience or bad news. Feverish and extremely restless with insomnia.
Sleepy on going to bed, but wakes in the early hours feeling overheated	Restless and uncomfortable from a stuffy bedroom or heavy bedcovers. Throws covers off but pulls them back on again when too chilly. Cannot find a comfortable position in bed. Hot flashes and night sweats. Weepy and in need of sympathy.
Depressed and exhausted with interrupted sleep	Tired and sleepy during the day but has difficulties falling asleep at night. Wakes early and cannot get back to sleep. Gets up feeling unrefreshed and deprived of rest. Headaches, nausea, and dizziness from tiredness.
Disturbed sleep after an emotional shock	Insomnia may date from a bereavement. Never refreshed by sleep, which is broken by recurring disturbing dreams. Limbs jerk when falling asleep.

Better for	Worse from	Remedy
Warmth Warm drinks Lying propped up in bed Moving about	Approach of night Cold surroundings Being alone Alcohol	Arsenicum album
As the day goes on Warmth Being left undisturbed Resting	On first waking Interrupted sleep Cold, drafty conditions Coffee Alcohol	Nux vomica

Cool surroundings
Fresh air
Loose nightwear
	On waking
	Warm, stuffy
	   surroundings
	Constricting
	   nightclothes or
	   bedcovers
		Lachesis

Fresh air Sweating After a sound sleep	At night Stuffy bedrooms Alcohol Extreme heat or chill	Aconite
Cool surroundings Fresh air Gentle movement Cool drinks Affection	Stuffy rooms Becoming chilled Keeping still First half of the night	Pulsatilla
Vigorous exercise Fresh air Warm bed Napping	Emotional strain Being sedentary Before a period	Sepia
Deep breathing Moving about Solitude	Shock Emotional stress Yawning	Ignatia

taking your whole medical history, emotional well-being, and physical symptoms into account.

Practical Self-Help

STIMULANTS

Cut down or cut out strong tea, coffee, and caffeinated soft drinks. Drinking regular and sizeable quantities of caffeine during the day leads to wakefulness at night, as well as palpitations (consciousness of a rapid heartbeat), jitteriness, and headaches. Change to coffee substitutes that do not contain caffeine, decaffeinated coffee (from a source that uses a natural filtering process rather than chemical solvents to remove the caffeine), or one of the many herb teas that are now available.

If you drink large quantities of strong coffee, cut down the amount you drink each day, rather than abruptly cutting it out. This is to avoid caffeine withdrawal, which can lead to severe headaches and a general feeling of unwellness.

PRACTICALITIES

Ensure that your curtains block out light adequately and that your bedroom is well ventilated so that it is neither stuffy nor chilly. Keep a towel, washcloth, a fresh nightdress or T-shirt, and a bowl of water on your bedside table if you are being disturbed by night sweats. If you have these items ready, you can sponge yourself down until you feel cooler, and dry yourself thoroughly to ensure that you do not become chilled. Having dry nightwear at hand avoids the disruption of getting up and rummaging around in the middle of the night for a nightdress.

RELAXATION

Try to avoid working late so that your mind has a chance to unwind and relax before sleep. Do something that you find soothing before you go to bed. This may be listening to a favorite piece of music, using a relaxation technique, meditating, or soaking in a warm (but not too hot) bath. Essential oils that encourage relaxation and rest include geranium, neroli, camomile, rose, and sandalwood.

If you are having a restless night, it is best to get up and drink a soothing cup of camomile tea or read until you feel more relaxed. Tossing and turning in bed is likely to make you feel more tense and anxious about not being able to sleep.

EXERCISE

Make time for a long walk in the fresh air each day, ideally in the evenings to help you relax. Other aerobic activities that may be helpful include cycling and swimming, especially if you feel stressed and tense during the day.

WEIGHT GAIN

In any discussion of desirable weight, it is wise to bear in mind that it is not necessarily positive or healthy for us to aim to weigh the same at fifty as we did in our twenties. As we approach menopause, the distribution of fat on our bodies changes, often settling on our waists, thighs, tops of our arms, and abdomens. Provided we feel comfortable with the minor changes, there is no reason to suppose that we must lose these few extra inches and squeeze into the clothes size we wore in our thirties in order to be healthy.

However, if we feel that we have put on an excessive amount of weight and that it is making us breathless, lethargic, and lacking in confidence and self-esteem, we need to stop the process before it becomes a health hazard. This is especially true if we suffer from diabetes, arthritis, high blood pressure, varicose veins or a prolapse, which can all be aggravated by being overweight.

To establish whether you are overweight, it is often best to

Typical Features	*General Symptoms*
Easily tired and clammy with persistent weight gain	Gains weight easily because of slow metabolism. May have symptoms of underactive thyroid gland: chilliness, constipation, and sluggishness. Craves sweets, eggs, and dairy foods other than milk.
Easy weight gain from overrich diet	Tends to be overweight with a poor circulation. Alternates between feeling chilly and having hot flashes. Because of irregularities of circulation, hands and feet are always chilly and may develop chilblains. Weepy and sad due to weight problems.
Tendancy to be overweight with fluid retention	Always chilly because of a sluggish circulation. Puffy swellings from fluid retention, especially around eyes. Although overweight, possibly poorly nourished with tendency to be anemic. Feels run down and catches frequent colds.
Weight problems with craving for salty foods	Fluid retention, especially before a period. Skin is dry with cold sores on lips. A preoccupation with weight may follow a period of stress or grief. Either severely underweight or overweight. Cravings for salt, fish, and milk and aversions to rich foods, bread, and fat.
"Pear shaped" accumulation of weight on abdomen, hips, and thighs	Unequal distribution of weight, with thin face and torso. Digestion is poor, with rumbling, gurgling, and excess wind. Bloated feeling, especially after eating. Quickly satisfied after a few mouthfuls of food, but hungry about an hour later.

Better for	Worse from	Remedy
Moderate temperatures Dry weather Constipation	Physical effort Going without food Standing for long periods of time Being chilled Before or after a period	Calc. carb.
Fresh, open air Gentle exercise Wearing loose-fitting clothes Cold food and drinks	Becoming too warm Stuffy rooms Resting in bed Rich or fatty foods	Pulsatilla

Warmth	Becoming chilled
	Eating
	Touch
	Cold weather
	Midmorning when
	  faintness and hunger
	  develop
		Kali. carb.

Fresh air Skipping meals Cool bathing Gentle exercise	Heat Direct sunlight Stuffy rooms Stress Sympathy Too much physical exertion	Natrum mur.
Warmth Loosening clothes Fresh air Exercise	Becoming chilled Cold foods and drinks Emotional stress Anticipating an event Being unoccupied	Lycopodium

follow your subjective impressions of how comfortable you feel, rather than tables or charts that calculate how much you should weigh according to your height. If you cannot run easily or climb a couple of flights of stairs without getting breathless, or if you feel uncomfortable and restricted regardless of what you wear, you may be overweight. If you are overweight and most of your fat is distributed around and above your waist rather than on your hips and thighs, there is evidence to suggest that you may be slightly more at risk of developing heart disease.

Homeopathic Help

If you are concerned about being overweight or have had difficulties losing weight, seeking homeopathic treatment can be an appropriate course of action. Homeopathic practitioners cannot offer an instant solution to weight problems, but they can offer helpful advice from a dietary perspective, as well as prescribing appropriate homeopathic medicines.

Because your homeopathic prescription will be chosen to match your symptoms as a whole, a tendency to have an inefficient or sluggish metabolism will be taken into account. Eating patterns and food cravings are also important symptoms, often guiding the homeopath to the most appropriate remedy. As a result, when homeopathic treatment is successful, patients often find they gradually reach their optimum weight, as their bodies begin to function in a more balanced way.

Because weight gain can often be a long-term or persistent symptom, this condition can be described as "chronic." As a result, it is best to seek professional help if you have a weight problem, rather than attempting to select an appropriate homeopathic remedy for yourself. A small number of potentially helpful homeopathic medicines are listed below to give you an impression of what is appropriate for use in this situation, rather than to encourage you to self-prescribe.

Practical Self-Help

EXERCISE

If you eat a basically healthy diet but feel that you are carrying an excessive amount of weight or keep gaining excess pounds, consider how physically active you are. Regular exercise (ideally of an aerobic nature which conditions your heart and lungs) is an essential way of stimulating your metabolism into more vigorous action. As a result, you will find that you burn up your daily food intake increasingly efficiently, with the added bonus of an equivalent improvement in energy production.

Don't be put off by the idea that exercising regularly results in an increased appetite; in fact the reverse is true. If you exercise on an empty stomach, you are likely to find that you feel quite satisfied once you rest after physical activity is over. Remember that you should never engage in vigorous physical exercise on a full stomach; always wait at least an hour or two after eating.

DIET

Take an honest look at your daily food intake and evaluate how nutritious it is. Foods to concentrate on include a wide range of fruit and vegetables (ideally eaten raw or lightly boiled or steamed to preserve essential nutrients), whole grains such as brown rice, pulses, seeds, unsalted and unroasted nuts, homemade high-fiber soups, live natural yogurt, poultry (without the skin), and fish (unbattered). Eat a large helping of salad with each main meal, and have at least four pieces of fruit each day. Drink five or six large glasses of mineral or filtered water each day, especially if you have any history of cystitis or kidney problems. If you are hungry between meals, opt for crudités of fresh, chopped raw vegetables in season, a piece of fruit, or rice cakes with a savory topping.

Foods to avoid include highly processed prepared meals, which usually have a high proportion of sodium as well as other additives and preservatives. These can severely aggravate a tendency toward fluid retention. Keep junk foods to a minimum, especially cakes, cookies, and puddings, which often include large quantities of white sugar and flour as well as fat. Dairy foods should be eaten sparingly; opt for varieties of cheese and milk that are lower in fat, such as Edam cheese and skimmed or semiskimmed milk. Keep your consumption of alcohol, coffee, and tea to a minimum, and cut out or greatly reduce your intake of foods that are high in saturated fat, such as bacon, beef, and pork, and snack foods such as potato chips.

Avoid crash dieting since this tends to aggravate a weight problem. If we go on a diet that allows us the minimum amount of calories per day, we initially lose weight rapidly, but within a short time our bodies get used to this restricted amount of food. Once this happens, our metabolisms slow down to accommodate the change in eating patterns, and we cease to lose any additional pounds. As soon as we go back to a normal eating pattern, we gain weight steadily because our metabolisms have become sluggish. An additional disadvantage to extreme dieting is that our bodies begin to break down and utilize protein from our bodies if we are not obtaining sufficient vital nutrients from our daily intake of food.

Try to eat when you are relaxed and have enough time to enjoy your food. If snacks are being eaten on the run, or if you eat while being distracted by reading or watching television, you are unlikely to feel satisfied by your meal. Also make a habit of eating two main meals, as well as breakfast and supper, each day rather than "grazing" or snacking frequently on foods that are low in nutrients and high in fat or sugar.

Be aware that we often eat out of habit or boredom, rather than because we are genuinely hungry. Try to eat only if you have hunger pangs and your body is sending signals that you are ready to enjoy a meal.

SELF-IMAGE
Be realistic about your ideal weight, and remember that it is unhealthy to strive for a body shape that is too thin after

menopause. The amount of fat our bodies hold in reserve has a direct effect on the amount of estrogen we produce. In other words, those who are underweight at menopause often find they suffer more adverse symptoms than those who have an average or slightly heavier body weight.

CIRCULATORY PROBLEMS

The condition of our circulatory system depends on the healthy functioning of our hearts, veins, and arteries. As we get older, our circulatory systems tend to work less efficiently, leading to common problems such as varicose veins, high or low blood pressure, athero-sclerosis (furring up of the walls of the arteries), or arteriosclerosis (hardening and narrowing of the artery walls). Although a tendency to have circulatory problems can be inherited, there are positive steps we can take at an early stage to condition and protect our circulatory systems.

This is especially important news for women. There is a low incidence of heart attacks and angina among premenopausal women, but the risk of heart disease rises steadily in the post-menopausal years as levels of estrogen production go down. We should be aware that this problem can develop after menopause and take positive action to maximize the condition of our hearts and lungs as early as possible.

Homeopathic Help

Homeopathic medicine provides a tremendous potential for the treatment of a range of circulatory problems. However, because of the often well-established or serious nature of these conditions, self-prescribing is not recommended. Help should be sought from a homeopathic practitioner, who will be trained to deal with the complicated aspects of case management in a situation of this kind. This is especially true if conventional medication is being taken, such as beta-blockers or ACE inhibitors for the treatment of high blood pressure (hypertension).

However, the following suggestions are all positive steps you can take to protect or improve the function of your circulatory system at the most fundamental level.

Practical Self-help

CHECKUPS
Have your blood pressure checked at regular intervals. Because of its symptomless nature, many of us do not realize we have high blood pressure until it is picked up during a routine investigation.

DIET
Certain foods have a reputation for protecting the circulatory system, and others are known to have an adverse effect. You may consider eating oily fish regularly, which helps to lower levels of a low-density form of cholesterol, called low-density lipoproteins (LDL). This type of cholesterol is thought to contribute to the furring up of the artery walls, unlike high-density lipoproteins (HDL), which protect the circulatory system. Other foods to include in your diet are those that are good sources of fiber, such as wholemeal bread, brown rice, fruit and vegetables, and pulses. As well as helping to prevent obesity, constipation, varicose veins, and hemorrhoids, fiber may have a beneficial effect in protecting us against heart disease. You may also want to include other low-fat sources of protein in your diet, such as poultry, meat, and fish. Use small amounts of cold-pressed virgin olive oil if you are baking or grilling food. Olive oil is a monounsaturated fat that is thought to have a beneficial effect on the circulatory system.

Avoid saturated fats that are solid at room temperature such as lard, and do not deep-fry your food, but opt for grilling and stir-frying instead. Use butter and cream very sparingly, and try to cut out red meat such as beef and pork. Be aware that many commercially prepared dishes may also include a large amount of saturated fat. Always check the proportions, which should be listed on the packaging.

If you have high blood pressure, avoid salt whenever possible since it is thought to contribute to the problem. Many fast foods and snacks such as potato chips and nuts include a high proportion of salt in their ingredients, and are best avoided if you are concerned about your blood-pressure levels. Use other flavorings in moderation to avoid blandness in your cooking; try garlic, powdered seaweeds, herbs such as oregano, and mild spices.

Make sure that you stay well below your unit allowance for alcohol consumption (fourteen units maximum per week), and cut out or vastly reduce your intake of stimulants such as strong coffee and tea or switch to decaffeinated versions. A unit of alcohol consists of a small glass of wine, a measure of spirits, or half a pint of beer.

Avoid foods that combine large quantities of sugar and fat, such as cakes, cookies, and chocolate.

Garlic is thought to have a beneficial effect on the circulatory system and should be included on a regular basis in the diet. However, if you find the odor unappealing, you can consider using an odorless supplement of concentrated garlic powder in tablet form. If your intake of oily fish is limited, you can also consider using fish oil supplements which are high in omega 3 fatty acids. Another excellent source of omega 3 fatty acids is linseed oil.

EXERCISE

Regular exercise conditions the heart and lungs and is an essential way of protecting and conditioning our circulatory systems. Regular, rhythmic, aerobic exercise such as brisk walking, swimming, and cycling works our heart muscle, thus encouraging a lowered pulse rate when resting and often helping to lower slightly raised blood pressure. Regular aerobic activity also helps reduce stress and muscular tension and may stimulate the production of estrogen (the hormone that protects us against heart disease in our fertile years).

RELAXATION

Use relaxation and visualization techniques, meditation, or autogenic training as a way of managing stress. Autogenic training is a stress-relieving therapy that involves the repetition of six simple phrases or exercises. Another technique is biofeedback, which uses machines to monitor a range of reactions to stress, such as changes in body temperature, brainwave patterns, and fluctuations in blood pressure. By becoming aware of these negative responses, it is possible to modify them by using a range of visualization, breathing, and relaxation techniques.

Techniques such as these, when combined with other posi-tive changes in lifestyle, can be enormously beneficial to people who suffer from high blood pressure. If you are unsure where to start, attending a well-taught yoga class can be a good way to learn basic relaxation and breathing techniques. If you are suffering from heart disease or high blood pressure, or if you are taking orthodox medication, you should mention this to your teacher before you begin your class.

SMOKING

If you smoke cigarettes, make serious efforts to cut down drastically or give it up altogether. It is now common knowledge that smoking increases our risk of heart disease, cancer of the lungs, and bronchitis. Tobacco smoking is now understood to be one of the principal causes of arteriosclerosis and atherosclerosis because it damages the walls of the arteries. Additional problems faced by smokers include a greater risk of high blood pressure, osteoporosis, an early menopause, increased difficulties with hot flashes, and premature skin aging.

OSTEOPOROSIS

One of the major problems facing us in our postmenopausal years is the risk of developing osteoporosis. In this condition, our bones progressively lose their density and strength and slowly become more brittle. Once this problem is well established, a relatively minor trauma such as jolting or jarring can result in a fracture. This is particularly dangerous for the elderly, since a fractured thigh bone, for example, can cause complications that can be fatal. One of the most common fractures that indicates a potential susceptibility to osteoporosis is a fracture of the wrist. This can occur as the result of a fall where a hand is instinctively held out for protection. Other common symptoms of osteoporosis include:

- severe pain or discomfort in the weight-bearing joints of the hips and knees or in the back;
- muscle spasms or weakness of the pelvic floor;
- limited or restricted movement in the chest and/or spine.

If this third condition is allowed to progress, a "dowager's hump" may occur. This is the characteristic stooped appearance that some elderly women develop, which leads to a substantial loss of height.

There are certain predisposing factors that may make us more vulnerable to developing osteoporosis. They include the following.

- An early menopause can increase the risk of osteoporosis, whether it is a result of a natural process or of surgical intervention, such as hysterectomy. Women who have had both ovaries removed are at greater risk than those who have one or both ovaries remaining.
- A history of eating disorders, with an attendant disruption or stopping of period pains, can predispose

61

us to osteoporosis. Since low body weight is associated with low estrogen production, extreme dieting during the teenage years, when bone density is being built up, can take its toll in the years following menopause.

- We may inherit a predisposition to develop osteoporosis. Those who have close female relatives suffering from this problem may also be at greater risk than those who do not.

- Using steroids may also result in increased problems with osteoporosis.

Homeopathic Help

Alternative methods of healing, such as homeopathy, have a great deal of positive input to offer in the debate about the prevention and treatment of osteoporosis. Homeopathic practitioners work from the basis that the majority of health problems are the result of disturbances in the smooth functioning of the body's self-healing, self-regulating, and renewing mechanisms. It is therefore quite appropriate to seek homeopathic advice when dealing with the problem of osteoporosis.

However, because of the serious nature of the problem, it is a condition that must be dealt with by consulting a skilled practitioner rather than attempting to self-prescribe. As well as selecting an appropriate homeopathic medicine after a detailed case analysis, your homeopath should be able to give you the most up-to-date advice on the changes you can make in your lifestyle to maximize your chances of positively managing the condition. Some of this essential advice is included in the self-help section below.

In any debate about osteoporosis, it is essential to discuss the pros and cons of hormone replacement therapy (HRT). This is the conventional medical treatment that is most likely to be offered to women who are worried about developing brittle bones in the years following menopause. Because of the importance of this issue, chapter 6 has been devoted to discussing the controversy surrounding the use of HRT. Within this chapter there is a section on the merits and demerits of HRT in the treatment of osteoporosis.

Practical Self-Help

EXERCISE

Keep as mobile as possible. An immobile or sedentary lifestyle encourages calcium to leach from our bones in the post-menopausal years, and keeping physically active is vital for maintaining healthy bone density. Regular weight-bearing exercise is one of the best tools we have at our disposal for protecting the strength and quality of our bones. It encourages the production of small amounts of estrogen, which protects our skeletal systems. Appropriate forms of weight-bearing exercise include brisk walking, cycling, and low-impact aerobics classes.

It is best to become active as early as possible, rather than waiting until long after menopause has passed us by, since we usually reach peak bone mass at around the age of thirty-five. However, it is never too late to become fit and active. If you are not attracted by jogging or aerobics classes, find a form of physical activity that you enjoy, and you may be surprised to find how much stamina and energy you will gain. Additional forms of exercise you might want to try include swimming, tennis, badminton, or squash. Be careful, however, not to overtax yourself, particularly when playing fast, competitive games like squash.

DIET

The quality of our diets before, during, and after menopause is essential in maintaining good bone density. Make sure you have a good supply of calcium-rich foods, remembering that there are excellent sources beyond the obvious dairy products such as milk, cheese, and yogurt. Dark green, leafy vegetables such as spinach and broccoli are rich in calcium, as well as nuts, seeds, fish, wholemeal bread, tofu, and dried fruit (especially figs). The average daily requirement of calcium for women who do not take HRT is 1,500 mg at the age of forty and 1,200 mg by the age of sixty.

If you are concerned about your calcium intake and feel you would benefit from extra calcium in supplement form, remember that it is best to take a combined calcium and magnesium formula. This is because the two minerals act in combination, and need to be balanced in a specific ratio in order to be utilized by the body. Although phosphorus is needed to enhance the absorption of calcium into our bones, too much of it will have the opposite effect, effectively promoting demineralization of our skeletal systems. Some foods, such as soft drinks, packet soups, and desserts, and processed cheeses and meats contain high quantities of phosphorus, and should be avoided or eaten infrequently in small quantities.

Consider supplementing your diet with vitamins C, D, and E. This may be appropriate if you feel that your diet is lacking in sufficient supplies of raw, fresh fruit and vegetables through the winter months, or if you do not spend much time out of doors (vitamin D is manufactured by the body provided we get sufficient daily exposure to daylight).

Although we must have protein to build and repair our bodies, an excess in the diet from animal sources such as red meat may aggravate osteoporosis.

Avoid regular caffeine and alcohol intake, since both are likely to aggravate osteoporosis.

SMOKING

Cigarette smoking is associated with an increased risk of osteoporosis. It diminishes estrogen production, and can contribute to an early menopause. (For more on the hazards of smoking, see "Circulatory Problems," p. 57.)

LOSS OF LIBIDO

From middle age onward, sexual responses begin to change for men as well as women. This does not necessarily mean that things have to change for the worse: quite the opposite can be true. Many of us will find that if these changes take place within the context of a balanced and healthy sex life, the freedom that comes from dispensing with contraception can be exhilarating. If we have relied on barrier methods of contraception such as a diaphragm or condom during our fertile years, many of us find that our sex lives become more spontaneous and enjoyable when these are no longer needed. This sense of freedom can also be enhanced by the increased privacy that comes when our children have grown up and are no longer inclined to interrupt an intimate moment.

However, menopause can be a time when sexual desire declines, and attendant problems may emerge. This situation often arises if we have sexual problems that have remained unresolved from an earlier phase of a relationship, or if we feel uneasy with or unconfident about our physical desirability. The latter can be a particular problem for those of us who have never felt at ease with our bodies and who may have a history of eating disorders.

The factors that contribute to a decline in libido can include an underlying tendency to depression, an aversion to sex because intercourse has become painful, or a general lack of energy and zest for life.

Homeopathic Help

Because the reasons for a decline in sex drive can be so varied, homeopathy has a great deal to offer in helping with the problem, because of its holistic and broad-ranging approach. To a homeopath, mental and emotional symptoms are as important as physical disorders. It is therefore the pattern formed by the individual's

Typical Features	*General Symptoms*
Loss of libido with indifference to sexual partner	Physically exhausted and depressed by family demands. Irritable with, or couldn't care less about, children and partner. Depressed, hopeless, and weepy when sex drive is low. Soreness, itchiness, and sensitivity of the vagina.
Aversion to sex due to painful dryness of vagina	A history of fluid imbalances, including water retention, and dry, cracked skin with cold sores. Genital area becomes sore and dry after menopause, with possible prolapse. Depressed and withdrawn, with dislike of physical affection.
Exhausted and tense after intercourse	Exceptionally chilly with marked fatigue, possibly due to anemia. Persistent fluid retention with puffy swellings under the eyes. Periods are heavy and flooding, with low back pain. Tense and hypersensitive to slightest touch or noise. Feels strung out, on edge, and unable to cope.
Sexual problems following surgery such as hysterectomy	Genital area may be very sensitive, with stinging, sharp pains on slightest touch. Persistent cystitis is worse from intercourse. Feelings of anger or resentment after invasive surgery.
Complete lack of interest in sex due to uterine prolapse	Gradual diminishing of previously high sex drive. Eventually feels worn out, depressed and very worried about general state of health. Alternates between euphoria and hopelessness. Feels prematurely old.

Better for	Worse from	Remedy
Vigorous exercise Fresh air After a nap Eating	Emotional demands Sitting quietly Before a period	Sepia
Cool bathing of sensitive areas Cool, fresh surroundings Skipping meals Being left alone	Emotional demands Sympathy Becoming overheated After a nap During or after a period	Natrum mur.
Warmth	Chill Eating Touch	Kali. carb.
Warmth Resting After eating	Sexual contact Emotional stress or anger Light touch Pressure	Staphysagria
	Physical effort Sexual contact	Agnus castus

symptoms as a whole that leads the homeopath to the selection of the most appropriate homeopathic prescription. A well-selected homeopathic medicine can give the body the energy boost it requires to stimulate vitality, lift depression, and regulate imbalances in bodily functions.

If your symptoms occur infrequently, are of recent onset, and are not severe, an occasional dose of an appropriate remedy selected from the table below may help a great deal. However, if you are depressed and taking conventional medication or suffer from severe or well-established physical symptoms such as vaginal dryness or soreness, it is best to consult a homeopath for a professional opinion. This is also the case if you need to continue taking a homeopathic medicine for an extended period in order to maintain an improvement.

Practical Self-Help

FATIGUE

If you feel your flagging libido is related to a general sense of lethargy and lack of vitality, see the advice included in the section "General Fatigue and Low Energy Levels" (p. 42). Just as a strong and healthy sex drive is intimately connected to having an abundance of energy and vitality, if we feel exhausted we are unlikely to have the necessary zest to enjoy a lively and fulfilling sex life. If we can rectify problems of diminishing energy levels, our physical relationships often measurably improve in quality.

DEPRESSION

Lack of interest in sex can be a common symptom of depression. If you have been feeling low for no apparent reason, and this feeling of sadness is accompanied by loss of appetite or diminishing interest in food, sleep disturbance, feeling anxious on waking, or low physical and mental energy, you may be suffering from depression. If this is the case, and you feel it has continued for some time without showing signs of improvement, you should seek a professional opinion from an alternative or conventional medical practitioner. You may also benefit from the advice given in chapter 3 in the section "Depression" (p. 35).

STRESS

Evaluate how much stress you have in your life. When tension builds, our interest in sex is often the first thing to suffer. If you feel that this is contributing to your problem, consider the following suggestions as strategies for coping with a stressful lifestyle.

- Investigate learning a relaxation or meditation technique to enable you to relax and unwind.
- Consider taking up a form of enjoyable exercise to provide an outlet for excess adrenaline.
- Avoid foods that make us more vulnerable to the adverse effects of stress. These include coffee, strong tea, caffeinated cola drinks, cigarettes, alcohol (especially spirits), and junk foods.
- If you suffer from painful muscular tension in your neck and shoulders, explore the benefits of a regular massage. If you don't have time for a full body treatment, most therapists will be happy to focus on a back and shoulder treatment.

SEX

A lack of interest in or aversion to intercourse may be related to physical discomfort or pain associated with lovemaking. These problems may be due to changes that occur after menopause, such as dryness or thinning of the vaginal wall, which can make intercourse very painful. Recurrent yeast infections or cystitis can also wreak havoc with our sex lives. Avoid using vaginal deodorants, and do not use soap to lather within the vaginal opening since this will only serve to further dry out the area. Use a lubricating jelly inside and around the opening of the vagina before intercourse, and do not rush foreplay. This can often be the most pleasurable part of lovemaking, and it also ensures that there is sufficient lubrication. Remember that regular and fulfilling sexual activity will help prevent vaginal dryness as we get older.

DIET

Include foods in your diet that are good sources of the minerals and vitamins that play a part in preserving a healthy libido. These include rich sources of zinc, which can be obtained from whole grains, sardines, herrings, oysters, seeds, nuts, and seafood. Also ensure that you have a regular intake of vitamins from the B complex. Niacin (vitamin B_3) is most important because it is associated with histamine production, which enhances sex drive. Niacin may be found in liver, kidney, mackerel, brown rice, cod, pulses, potatoes, and eggs. If you have any concern about obtaining the full range of B vitamins from your diet, consider taking a B complex supplement.

EXERCISE

Exercising and toning the muscles of your vaginal floor can heighten sexual pleasure for both partners. We can locate these muscles by stopping and starting the flow of urine as we pass water. Consciously tightening and relaxing these muscles leads to enhanced control of this area.

OTHER FACTORS

Remember that there are certain orthodox drugs that may diminish sexual desire. These include drugs that lower high blood pressure, such as beta-blockers, some antidepressants, and antihistamines. Many women may also experience diminished sexual pleasure and desire after a hysterectomy, especially if their ovaries have been removed.

Counseling

If you feel that your sex life is suffering because of unresolved problems between you and your partner, you could benefit from counseling.

5

Homeopathy and Common Physical Symptoms

If you consult a homeopath, you will discover that they put a tremendous emphasis on the links between physical, emotional, and mental symptoms. Within this framework, the patterns formed by physical symptoms often begin to make sense when seen from the perspective of emotional stresses or traumas that may have been present before the physical symptoms set in. For instance, a mysterious skin eruption can often emerge after excessive emotional strain, too harsh or pressured conditions at work, or a period of indifferent or poor quality health.

Although this type of crossover effect is especially true of menopausal problems, where emotional and physical symptoms can seem firmly interlinked, there are certain difficulties that we can identify as primarily affecting our sense of physical well-being.

In this chapter you will find a survey of these conditions, giving positive advice from a homeopathic and general self-help perspective. As always, consult the practical information given in chapter 2. If you are familiar with the instructions given in this section, you are most likely to experience a positive outcome.

HOT FLASHES AND NIGHT SWEATS

Although there are certain common features to hot flashes, the severity, duration, and amount of distress associated with the problem can vary enormously. Some of us may dread the onset of a hot flash because of the embarrassment it causes and the emotional and physical distress it leaves in its wake, while others of us may scarcely be aware of a problem.

The widespread nature of these symptoms has been made clear by a recent American survey that suggested that approximately 75 percent of postmenopausal women will experience hot flashes, with 45 percent seeking medical treatment to help deal with the problem. If we accept that the majority of us stand a good chance of experiencing hot flashes when we approach or go through menopause, it makes a great deal of sense to be aware of how we first identify that this is our problem and how we can support ourselves using simple and effective self-help measures.

One of the factors that may contribute to the severity of the hot flashes experienced is the rate and abruptness with which estrogen production and ovulation ceases. If this process is relatively slow and gradual, with a resulting slow reduction in our periods, there is a good chance that menopausal symptoms such as hot flashes may be minimal. On the other hand, if the process is more abrupt, the resulting symptoms are likely to be more severe.

The following list gives a broad description of some of the common sensations associated with hot flashes.

- There may be an unpredictable and abrupt feeling of warmth or heat, which may radiate upward from the waist to the neck and face. The skin may look flashed and feel burning hot to the touch. This sensation of heat may be accompanied or quickly followed by a profuse sweat, which leaves the skin feeling cool, clammy, and shivery.
- Many of us experience a feeling of foreboding, anxiety, or general unease a second or two before a flash sets in. Others may wake during the night just before a flash or night sweat occurs.

Typical Features	*General Symptoms*
Hot flashes that occur at night or on waking	Negative reaction to temperature change: head feels hot but lower half of body feels cold. Waves of heat surge through body in a wavelike motion. Tense, agitated, and talkative with anxiety. Finds any pressure around neck (scarf or tight sweater) unbearable.
Lack of stamina with tendency to sweat on least exertion	Hot flashes with even slight physical exertion or when under emotional strain. Internal sensation of heat, and skin feels clammy and sweaty. Feels cold and chilly as soon as activity stops. Becomes anxious and insecure easily, especially when observed.
Easy flushing with craving for fresh air	Distressed and feels on the verge of collapse with flashes of heat. Although skin feels ice-cold and clammy to the touch, internal sensations of burning heat. Hot flashes may be brought on by eating spicy food or drinking wine.
Flushing with bright red, dry skin	Violent hot flashes start suddenly, with skin that is characteristically bright red and dry to the touch. Skin is so hot it radiates heat. Sweats on parts of body that are covered. Irritable and oversensitive to sensory stimulation.
Flashes of heat with marked anxiety	Hot flashes often follow eating or drinking hot food or drinks. Feels as though whole body has been dipped in hot water. Burning sensations with hot sweats on head and hands.
Alternating hot and cold sweats with marked depression	Easily exhausted and worn out from slight effort. Flashes move upward with dizziness on waking. Sweats are very heavy at night resulting in exhaustion through the day. Very apathetic, lethargic, and depressed.
Heat and burning with dry or moist skin	Severe hot flashes with flushed, dry skin. Flashes feel much worse for warm covering, especially when in bed. Must put feet outside bedcovers to get comfortable.

Homeopathy and Common Physical Symptoms

Better for	Worse from	Remedy
Fresh air Movement Cool places Peace and quiet	Stuffy rooms Exposure to sunlight Rapid temperature changes Tight clothing At night or after sleep	Lachesis
Moderate warmth Resting	Becoming chilled or damp Cold drafts Sudden changes of weather Before a period	Calc. carb.
Cool, fresh air Being fanned	Hot, stuffy rooms After eating Alcohol Movement	Carbo veg.
Resting Keeping still Moderate warmth	Exposure to cold air Drafts Movement Sensory stimulation	Belladonna
Reassurance Being touched Moderate warmth	Being alone Putting hands in cold water Evenings	Phosphorus
Fresh air Brisk walking Eating a little	Before a period Sitting still Emotional demands	Sepia
Avoiding exposure to extreme heat or cold Resting	Warm, stuffy rooms After bathing Standing for too long Waking from sleep	Sulphur

- We may have a general difficulty in dealing with temperature changes, with an intolerance of extreme heat or extreme cold.

Homeopathic Help

The following table will give an overview of some of the most commonly indicated homeopathic medicines for the relief of hot flashes. If your symptoms are happening infrequently and are mild in nature, you may find that an occasional dose of the appropriate remedy will improve the situation considerably.

However, if you suffer from frequent and severe hot flashes that do not respond positively to what appears to be a well-indicated remedy, you should seek professional help from a trained homeopath. This does not mean that you are suffering from symptoms that are unusually difficult to treat, but it is an indication that more deep-acting (constitutional) homeopathic treatment is required to return your whole system to balance.

Practical Self-Help

CLOTHING

Wear loose, layered, comfortable clothing that is unrestricting around your neck and waist and under your arms. Wear natural fibers and avoid synthetics like polyester. If you start to feel hot, you can take off the top layer until you feel cool enough to replace it. This way you can adapt quickly to your surroundings with the minimum of embarrassment and fuss.

EXERCISE

Regular exercise will benefit your circulatory system and discourage hot flashes. Ideal forms of exercise include brisk walking, tennis, running, and swimming.

Avoid or cut down smoking, spicy foods, salt, coffee, tea, chocolate and sugary foods, and sweetened drinks. Eat as many whole foods as possible (grains, pulses, raw fruits and vegetables) and consider supplementing with vitamins C, B complex, and E.

RELAXATION
Explore relaxation and breathing techniques that can help you cope with palpitations and feelings of panic during a hot flash.

PRACTICALITIES
If you suffer from night sweats, keep your bedroom cool and well ventilated, avoid synthetic nightclothes and bed linen, and have some lukewarm (not ice-cold) water at hand. You can sponge yourself with the tepid water if you feel feverish, enabling your skin to cool down as quickly as possible.

FLUID RETENTION

Many of us will be familiar with the symptoms of fluid retention associated with our monthly cycles. They can include a sensation of tightness or swelling in the waist, fingers, or feet. In addition, the breasts may be very painful, enlarged, and tender. Fluid retention can also be responsible for the extra pounds of weight we may gain before a period, and the general sense of fatigue or sluggishness that can also occur at the same time.

Women who suffer from premenstrual syndrome often experience fluid retention as one of the many symptoms associated with the disorder. It is worth noting that if we are subject to PMS in our twenties and thirties, these symptoms may become more severe as we approach menopause.

Typical Features	*General Symptoms*
Restlessness and fidgeting with fluid retention	Puffy, swollen breasts that are excruciatingly sensitive to touch or movement. Cool air and cool water locally applied are very soothing. Tissues around eyes may also look puffy or swollen.
Exhausted and cold-sensitive with fluid retention	Craves warmth, which temporarily soothes discomfort. General puffy swellings, especially noticeable around upper eyelids.
Fluid retention with marked thirst and craving for salt	Everything is worse before or after a period: headaches, depression, and hot flashes. Hair and skin are dry with a tendency to split or crack. Withdrawn, brooding, and antisocial due to fluid retention.
Fluid retention with lack of appetite and constant thirst	Constantly cold and restless with a dislike of sitting still for too long. Burning sensations with fluid retention and severe mood swings. Although food tastes insipid, generally feels better for eating.
Fluid retention with very painful breasts that are worse for slightest movement	Symptoms develop slowly over a few days. Although sensitive to the slightest movement or touch, firm pressure gives relief (e.g. supporting breasts with hands when running downstairs). Thirsty for cold drinks.
Fluid retention with general tendency to gain weight	Constant hunger and cravings for dairy foods and sweets with fluid retention. Constantly chilly and exhausted with aversion to exercise of any kind. Generalized puffy swellings in breasts, feet, and fingers.

Homeopathy and Common Physical Symptoms

Better for	Worse from	Remedy
Movement or exercise Removing clothes Contact with cool air Bathing with cool water	Lack of exercise Touch or pressure Warmth in any form	Apis (contraindicated if pregnancy is suspected)
Warmth	Cold in any form Touch Pressure Lying on painful area Coffee	Kali. carb.
Cool bathing Fresh, open air Gentle exercise Being left alone	Stuffy, warm rooms After sleep or resting Emotional stress Sympathy	Natrum mur.
While eating Evenings Resting	Mental strain Missing meals Exposure to cold drafts	Anacardium
Keeping as still as possible Firm pressure Lying on painful area Cool air and drinks	Light touch Any movement Warmth in any form	Bryonia
Warmth	Cold in any form Damp Before and during periods Making a physical effort	Calc. carb.

Homeopathic Help

If you suffer from a general tendency toward mild fluid retention before your periods, you will find that taking the homeopathic medicine that most closely matches your individual symptoms should promote a noticeable improvement. Once this improvement has set in, it is important to stop taking the selected remedy. A positive response is an indication that the necessary stimulation has been given to your body to deal with the problem itself, and any extra stimulation is unnecessary and may be counterproductive.

However, if you experience fluid retention within the context of severe PMS, it is recommended that you seek professional help in order to deal with the problem at a fundamental level.

Practical Self-Help

DIET

Avoid food and drinks that have a reputation for making fluid retention worse. These include coffee, tea, alcohol, salt, dairy foods, and convenience foods. Concentrate on raw, whole foods if you feel fluid retention developing, and exploit the diuretic (fluid-eliminating) qualities of fresh parsley.

Instead of cutting down on the amount of fluid you drink, make sure that you have six or eight large glasses of filtered water daily. This will encourage your kidneys to work more efficiently, flashing out toxins and discouraging the development of water-logged tissues.

Eat a high-fiber diet to avoid constipation, which can add to the discomfort of fluid retention, especially around the waist and abdomen.

If breast discomfort is severe, an oil of evening primrose supplement may be helpful.

EXERCISE

Make sure you exercise regularly two or three times a week. Regular, rhythmic, muscular movement stimulates the efficient functioning of the lymph system. Healthy functioning of this system is essential for the elimination of toxins from the body.

HEAVY PERIODS

As we approach menopause it can be alarming to find that periods that were previously regular and undistressing become uncharacteristically heavy, irregular, or painful. They may become totally unpredictable, with intervals between bleeding either shortening or lengthening. The nature of the flow itself may also change from moderate bleeding toa flooding or gushing that we find difficult to manage with sanitary protection.

If you experience heavy bleeding premenopausally, it is likely that your GP will want to check that this is due to expected changes at this time, rather than any other condition that has developed, such as endometriosis, fibroids, or polyps. Once it is established that your changed menstrual patternis due to premenopausal adjustments in hormone levels (such as low levels of progesterone), the problem is likely to clear spontaneously.

Homeopathic Help

Homeopathic treatment has a tremendous amount to offer in managing the distress that can be a part of a changed menstrual pattern. If you find that your monthly flow has recently been increasing, one of the following remedies may help a great deal in regulating the flow. However, do remember to notify your GP of any marked change in the regularity or intensity of your periods. Also consider seeking professional homeopathic advice if symptoms are severe or well established and seem beyond the scope of self-prescribing.

Typical Features	*General Symptoms*
Bright red, clotted, gushing flow	Severe dragging, cramping pains before period with general sense of congestion. Irritable and restless with pains. Skin is hot, bright red, dry and flushed during the pains.
Dizziness, anxiety, and exhaustion from blood loss	Apathetic and indifferent from low energy reserves. Tiredness leads to weepiness, depression, and headaches with heavy sensations behind eyes. Very heavy, bright red, clotted flow.
Persistent heavy bleeding with severe backache	Anemic and chilly with backache and pain in base of spine before and during periods. Painful areas feel unbearably cold. Exhausted with bleeding: even speaking is too much of an effort. Fluid retention and bloated abdomen.
Frequent, heavy periods with vertigo and anaemia	Heavy bleeding with faintness and buzzing in ears. Flow is dark, heavy and very clotted. Although chilly, bouts of shivering alternate with hot flashes. Exhausted, irritable, touchy, and antisocial due to blood loss.
Distressing pains with very dark, clotted flow	Pains relieved as soon as flow begins. Depression, mood swings, and severe left-sided headaches before flow begins. Hot flashes, faintness, and palpitations with flooding. Strong aversion to heat and constricting clothes.
Terrible nausea with bright red, heavy bleeding	Possible steady bleeding or alternation between oozing and gushing. Craves cool air when nauseated or faint. Severe nausea is much worse from movement of any kind.

Better for	Worse from	Remedy
Warmth Resting semi-erect in bed	Physical effort Jarring motion Lying flat	Belladonna
Massage Reassurance Warmth	Exertion Exposure to cold Excitement	Phosphorus
Warmth Leaning forward	Exposure to cold drafts Cold in any form Pressure Touch Lying on painful area	Kali. carb.
Warmth Sleep Rest Firm pressure	Making an effort Exposure to cold Fresh air At night	China
Onset of period Cool drinks Fresh, open air Eating Gentle exercise	Exposure to extreme heat or cold Stuffy, airless rooms Hot bathing Cold drafts Before period begins After sleep	Lachesis
Keeping as still as possible Closing eyes Fresh, cool air	Movement Eating Extreme heat or cold	Ipecac

Practical Self-Help

ANEMIA

If you suspect you may be anemic (lacking in iron), check for the following symptoms, which are common features of anemia:

- exhaustion or persistent tiredness;
- palpitations;
- breathlessness;
- pale complexion.

DIET

To protect against iron deficiency, include regular helpings of the following foods in your diet: wholemeal bread, nuts, seeds, green vegetables, oatmeal, molasses, pulses, fish, and eggs. Avoid dairy foods, strong tea, coffee, and alcohol.

EXERCISE

Boost your circulatory system by taking regular, vigorous exercise such as walking or cycling in the fresh air.

VAGINAL DRYNESS AND DISCOMFORT

One of the most commonly experienced and distressing problems we may encounter after menopause is vaginal dryness. Although this troublesome symptom can cause unhappiness for many women and their sexual partners, there is a great deal that can be done to ease the situation and restore the pleasure that is at the center of a satisfying sex life.

In order to find strategies for coping, it is necessary to under-stand why vaginal dryness becomes a problem after menopause. When we are young, sexual arousal results in speedy rushes of blood to the breasts, clitoris, vagina, and vulva. This increase in blood flow helps to keep the mucous membranes of the vagina supple, while estrogen levels will maintain the elasticity of the vagina. After menopause, blood does not flow as readily to these areas as it did in our youth, and decreasing estrogen levels lead to fragile vaginal tissues that are more susceptible to irritation and infection. Resulting problems can include:

- persistent irritation, itching, and recurrent vaginal infections;
- pain during sexual intercourse;
- if the situation is very severe, extreme dryness leading to cracking and bleeding of the vaginal walls.

Although this picture may sound bleak, there is a great deal that can be done to protect against the problem by making positive use of practical self-help measures and appropriate homeopathic remedies.

Homeopathic Help

In the following table you will find a survey of the homeopathic medicines that have a particular affinity with problematic sensitivity and dryness of the vaginal area. In combination with positive self-help measures, effective homeopathic prescribing can have a vital role to play in easing the problems associated with vaginal dryness.

Practical Self-Help

TOILETRIES
Avoid strongly scented soaps, foam baths, and vaginal sprays or deodorants. All of these can aggravate vaginal irritation and dryness.

Typical Features	**General Symptoms**
Dryness and soreness that are much worse for movement	General dryness of skin and mucous membranes. Stubborn constipation associated with a dry, large stool that is difficult to pass. Pains are sore or stitching and very sensitive to slight touch or movement. Irritable and anxious with pains.
Vaginal irritation with hot flashes and anxiety	Tension and anxiety lead to digestive problems, including heartburn, indigestion, excess wind, and diarrhea. Poor circulation, with dry, flaky skin, especially on scalp.
Vaginal discomfort with stitching, stinging pains	Symptoms are often experienced after a hysterectomy, especially where there is a lot of suppressed anger and resentment about having had surgery. Genital area is painfully sensitive and itchy.
Vaginal dryness with severe itching that is worse from walking	Complete aversion to sexual activity due to tenderness of vagina. Vaginal discomfort may be made worse by prolapse of womb or bladder. Very depressed and generally lacking in libido and "get up and go."

Better for	Worse from	Remedy

Cool water, locally applied
Keeping as still as possible
	Warmth
	First movement after
	    keeping still, e.g. rising
	    from a sitting position
		Bryonia

Moderate warmth Loosening clothes Being occupied	Becoming chilled or overheated Physical overexertion	Lycopodium
Resting Warmth	Slight touch or contact Sexual contact Emotional stress	Staphysagria
Vigorous movement Fresh, open air Resting in bed Having a nap Firm pressure	Emotional demands Touch Sitting still	Sepia

SEX

Taking plenty of time for foreplay during lovemaking can help enormously in minimizing pain from vaginal dryness. Using a water-based lubricating jelly can also be invaluable in easing discomfort and soreness.

Regular sexual activity has an important role to play in maintaining lubrication of the genital area. Reaching orgasm, with its attendant increased blood flow and muscular contractions, can play an essential role in maintaining the elasticity and lubrication of the vaginal area.

CLOTHING

If you suffer from vaginal itchiness and irritation, avoid wearing tights, jeans, or nylon underwear for extended periods. All of these will create a warm, humid environment that provides the optimum condition for the growth of vaginal infections. Opt instead for loose-fitting cotton panties, which create cooler, more ventilated conditions. If you love wearing jeans or leggings during the day, make sure you spend the evenings wearing something loose and airy.

TOPICAL APPLICATIONS

If you experience general soreness, apply Calendula cream to the painful area. This provides a soothing, topical application that can be used as often as required. Bathing with a *diluted* solution of Hypercal™ tincture (a mixture of Calendula and Hypericum) can also be invaluable in providing speedy relief to painful tissues.

Apply liberal amounts of live, natural, plain yogurt to the vaginal area if it feels itchy and irritated.

URINARY PROBLEMS AND STRESS INCONTINENCE

Because of the proximity of the vagina and the lower urinary tract to each other, both areas can be adversely affected by a reduction in estrogen levels after menopause. As a result, many of us may experience a range of potential problems in this area during menopause when estrogen levels are reduced. Possible difficulties include:

- a frequent and urgent desire to urinate, even if there is very little urine to be passed;
- discomfort or burning sensations on passing urine;
- leakage or dribbling of urine when running, carrying heavy weights, sneezing, coughing, or laughing.

These problems can be further compounded if a prolapse occurs. This condition results when the uterine ligaments supporting the womb begin to lose their tone and sag. When this occurs (often as a result of childbirth), the womb can descend to the point where it may protrude from the vagina. Other organs that might also begin to droop include the urethra (urethrocele), bladder (cystocele), and rectum (rectocele). Common symptoms of prolapse include:

- persistent backache;
- vaginal irritation from protrusion of the womb into the vagina;
- difficulties with penetration during intercourse as a result of the descended cervix (neck of the womb).

Homeopathic Help

Appropriately prescribed homeopathic medicines can have a very positive role to play in easing the discomfort and distress of urinary problems. Persistent urging and stress incontinence can respond well to homeopathy if the problem is due to declining muscle tone. However, if you suffer from persistent or severe symptoms, or if you suspect that the problem may be due to a bladder infection,it is advisable to seek professional advice.

Typical Features	*General Symptoms*
Poor muscle tone with general aches and pains	Heavy or constricted sensations in womb. Overwhelming need to lie down, with difficulty in making the slightest effort. Depressed and exhausted with prolapse of womb.
Urinary problems date from pregnancy or childbirth	Persistent stress incontinence when coughing, sneezing or laughing. Frequent sensation of needing to pass water must be acted on straight away or urine is passed involuntarily. Weepy and in need of sympathy when symptoms are severe.
Dragging, bearing-down sensations with slow flow of urine	Symptoms of prolapse of womb following childbirth. These include back-ache and a feeling as though everything were about to fall out of vagina. Sits with legs crossed to feel more secure and comfortable. Very depressed, exhausted, and indifferent with aversion to sexual partner.
Stinging and burning when passing concentrated urine	Constant feeling of not having emptied bladder completely. Discomfort during and after passing urine. Symptoms are aggravated by intercourse. Angry, irritable, and snappy with discomfort.
Slow-developing symptoms with unconscious passage of urine	Stress incontinence is worse from coughing or sneezing. Urine is passed involuntarily at night. Raw, sore, or tearing pains on urination, leaving affected area very sensitive to touch. Symptoms bring a general feeling of unwellness.
Excessive vaginal dryness with stress incontinence when coughing or walking	Low back pain that feels better for firm support in hollow of back. Flow of urine is slow to start. Aversion to intercourse due to discomfort in vagina. Withdrawn, depressed, and introverted when symptoms are severe.

Homeopathy and Common Physical Symptoms

Better for	Worse from	Remedy
Fresh air Stimulants Passing urine	Effort Being overheated Exposure to cold drafts	Gelsemium
Pressure Gentle movement Cool in general Fresh air Sympathy and attention After a good cry	At night Lying flat on the back Sitting or lying still Warm, stuffy rooms Feeling neglected	Pulsatilla
Pressure Warmth After a nap	Standing Walking Emotional demands	Sepia
Resting Warmth	Touch Sexual contact Pressure Early morning	Staphysagria
In bed Warmth	Becoming chilled or damp Movement Bathing Coffee	Causticum
Gentle movement Cool, fresh air Firm pressure Sitting with legs crossed	Overexertion Lying down Sleep Walking Coughing Becoming overheated	Natrum mur.

Practical Self-Help

EXERCISE

Do regular pelvic floor exercises to tighten the muscles in this area. These movements are very simple and involve contracting and relaxing your muscles while urinating, so that the flow stops and starts according to the number of contractions you choose to do. Once you are familiar with the sensation and location of these muscles, you can choose to do a series of pelvic floor exercises whenever it is convenient. Toning up these muscles also gives us the added bonus of increased vaginal control and sensation during lovemaking.

DIET

If you have a weight problem, embark on a sensible weight-loss plan. This should involve regular exercise to speed up your metabolic rate (the rate at which you burn up your food and convert it into energy) as well as dietary changes. Instead of crash dieting, eat large quantities of green vegetables, fruit, pulses, and grains. If you are not motivated to be vegetarian, concentrate on low-fat, easily digestible forms of protein such as fish or poultry (avoiding the skin). Avoid sweetened drinks, cakes, cookies, convenience foods, salt, snack foods such as potato chips and salted nuts, alcohol, coffee, tea, and large helpings of dairy foods. Eat plenty of fiber to avoid constipation, which can aggravate a prolapse.

Drink plenty of filtered water daily to guard against bladder infections or irritation. If you feel there is any suggestion of discomfort that may be due to a low-grade infection, drink cranberry juice at regular intervals (every hour for the first three to four hours). Drinking cranberry juice is an effective way of making your urine more alkaline, thus ensuring that it is less painful or irritating to pass. Also avoid any food or drink that may aggravate the problem. These include coffee, tea, alcohol, and sugary foods or drinks.

SMOKING

If you have a persistent smoker's cough, investigate ways of giving up smoking. Seek help, support, and advice from friends who are ex-smokers. Specific therapies that may help include counseling, hypnotherapy, acupuncture, and homeopathy. If a partner smokes, a compromise needs to be reached—perhaps restricting smoking to certain parts of the house—so that the problem of passive smoking can be overcome.

OTHER FACTORS

Avoid standing for long periods of time and put your feet up whenever possible.

Never put off urinating because you are too busy to do so until later. This can encourage infection to develop and can contribute to general discomfort. Each time you urinate, make sure you empty your bladder as completely as possible.

CYSTITIS

Although cystitis can occur at any time in our lives, the post-menopausal years can trigger an intensification of the problem. This is due to the key role that the hormone estrogen plays in maintaining healthy, infection-resistant urinary organs. Once hormone levels begin to fluctuate and fall, there is a general tendency for the tissues of these organs to become thinner and less able to combat infection.

Common symptoms of cystitis include the following:

- a constant desire to urinate with accompanying pains, which may vary from a general sense of discomfort to severe pains in the lower abdomen;
- very little urine passed at a time: often just a few drops of concentrated urine;

Typical Features	General Symptoms
Violent, abrupt onset of cystitis with fever	Sudden onset of pain and urgency which feel much worse for moving around. Urine may be bloody. Restless and feverish with red, hot, dry skin. Drowsy but cannot sleep.
Urgent need to pass concentrated, stinging urine	Thirstless with cystitis. Tissues around eyes look puffy and water-logged. Restless, fidgety, and irritable when feeling ill.
Abrupt onset of violent symptoms with terrible burning sensations	Exhausted and shivery with cystitis symptoms. Frequent, urgent need to urinate. Severe sharp or burning pains occur before, during, and after urination. Pains may travel to kidneys.
Cystitis that follows drinking an excess of coffee or alcohol	Feeling unwell follows overindulgence or overuse of medication such as painkillers. Burning or itching sensations when urinating. Constant discomfort with general sensitivity to cold. Very irritable when feeling ill.
Cystitis with slow-flowing urine	Generally sore, bloated, and uncomfortable in abdomen. Needs to loosen clothing to get comfortable. Pains in back and sides before urinating.
Icy coldness, restlessness, and anxiety with cystitis	Terrible burning pains that are soothed by warmth. Nausea or diarrhea with general feeling of unwellness. Cannot keep still. Hypersensitive to pain, noise, or the smell of food. Terribly anxious and distressed when ill.
Cystitis that follows a chill after overheating or becoming damp	Constant, urgent need to urinate. Fears passing urine involuntarily if there is the slightest delay. Discomfort remains after urinating and is worse for lying on the back. Very tearful and in need of consolation when ill.
Constant burning sensation that remains after urination	Terrible burning sensation, passing concentrated urine. Very thirsty for ice-cold drinks. Urine contains traces of blood. Very anxious.

Homeopathy and Common Physical Symptoms

Better for	Worse from	Remedy
Resting Warm rooms Sitting propped-up Keeping as still as possible	Movement Stimulation Light Noise	Belladonna
Contact with cool air Fresh air Applying cool compresses Movement Uncovering	Becoming heated Warm bathing Touch Lying down At night	Apis
Warmth At night	Motion Touch Drinking coffee	Cantharis
Warmth Sleep Resting As the day goes on Being left in peace	Exposure to cold drafts Stimulants Broken sleep Eating Mornings	Nux vomica
Fresh air Warm drinks Distraction	Becoming overheated Exposure to chill Stress In the afternoons	Lycopodium
Warmth Sips of warm drinks Hot water bottle applied to painful area Sitting propped up in bed	Exposure to cold Being alone Alcohol Cold drinks As the night goes on	Arsenicum album
Cool, fresh air Gentle exercise Company Sympathy Cold drinks	Sitting still At night Becoming overheated	Pulsatilla
Sleep Reassurance Physical contact Warmth	Exposure to cold Evenings Being alone Overexcitement	Phosphorus

- burning sensations before, during, or after urination;
- blood-stained urine in severe cases.

Homeopathic Help

Swift and accurate homeopathic prescribing can be a godsend in an acute bout of cystitis. For the most positive results it is best to catch the symptoms early, ideally at the first sign of discomfort. If you select the appropriate homeopathic medicine that matches your individual symptoms most closely, you should find that your symptoms are relieved within a few hours. However, if any of the following occurs, you should seek professional help:

- pain in the kidneys;
- nausea, vomiting or high temperature;
- blood-stained urine;
- persistent symptoms that do not improve from self-help measures.

Practical Self-Help

FLUIDS

Make sure that you drink enough filtered water each day to flash your kidneys and bladder regularly: ideally about five to six glasses each day. Don't be misled by thinking that increasing your tea or coffee intake is providing an adequate substitute for boosting your overall fluid intake. Unfortunately, both these drinks have a diuretic effect on the body, encouraging it to eliminate increased amounts of liquid.

At the first twinge of discomfort, drink a glass of cranberry juice every hour, continuing until the pain has eased.

Barley water also has a reputation for decreasing urine acidity. You can make your own by simmering pearl barley in a pan of water and straining off the liquid. Discard the barley and put the strained water in the fridge to cool. You can drink this liquid every hour until the inflammation and pain ease. Commercially prepared varieties of barley water are best avoided since they contain sugar and citrus fruit juice which contribute to increased acidity.

HYGIENE

You can discourage bladder and kidney infections by always making sure that you urinate when you feel the natural urge, rather than putting it off until later. Also ensure that you empty your bladder completely each time.

After a bowel movement, always wipe from front to back, rather than back to front. This simple measure will discourage the spreading of bacteria from the rectum and anus along the perineum to the urinary organs.

TOILETRIES

Use gently formulated, nonabrasive bath foams or soaps rather than strongly scented products. The latter may trigger or aggravate irritation and discomfort in the delicate tissues around the urogenital area.

ARTHRITIS

Although arthritis and general difficulties with mobility used to be seen as an inevitable part of the process of getting older, we are witnessing an increasing modification of these ideas. The generation that is currently moving into middle age has been better educated about the role that exercise and a healthy diet play in keeping fit than any previous generation. By being better informed about the factors that give us a good chance of keeping mobile, sturdy, flexible joints well into middle age, we are likely to face the challenge of these years with a much more positive outlook.

Common symptoms of osteoarthritis (the form of arthritis associated with the wear and tear of getting older) include pain, stiffness, or swelling in the large weight-bearing joints such as the hips, knees, and ankles. The pain and discomfort may come and go at irregular intervals, depending on temperature, humidity, and general weather conditions.

Rheumatoid arthritis commonly affects the small joints of the wrists, fingers, toes, ankles, heels, and the arch of the foot. It can happen at any age (it is called Stills disease in children), and may be preceded by a flulike illness. Joints characteristically feel hot, stiff, and swollen, and may look red and inflamed. Additional symptoms may include dry eyes and mouth, circulatory problems such as cold hands, chest problems, and swollen glands.

Homeopathic Help

Depending on the severity of the problem, homeopathy has an enormous amount to offer in helping the pain and general discomfort associated with joint problems. This help can be provided either in the form of an occasional dose of the appropriate remedy to minimize the discomfort of an acute (short-lived surfacing of symptoms) bout of joint pain, or from a professional source for more deep-seated, long-term, or severe problems.

If your symptoms are mild and occur infrequently, you may find speedy and prompt relief is provided by self-prescribing the appropriate remedy that corresponds most to your individual symptoms from the following table. However, if you need to take your remedy on a long-term basis to keep your symptoms stable, or if a well-indicated remedy does not promote a general improvement in your condition, you should seek professional help.

Practical Self-Help

DIET

Certain foods have the reputation of making joint problems worse. These include red meat; sugary cakes; and carbonated drinks that are heavily sweetened; convenience foods that contain a high proportion of refined (white) flour or sugar; coffee, tea, and alcohol; citrus fruits such as oranges, grapefruit, and lemons; and vegetables that belong to the nightshade family, including potatoes, tomatoes, green peppers, and eggplants. (The nightshade family is the name commonly given to *Solanaceae*, which also includes belladonna—deadly nightshade—and tobacco.)

Change your eating patterns in order to take the toxic load off your joints. Eat as many raw fruits and vegetables as possible (excluding the items mentioned above) by incorporating a large salad with your main meals each day, and having fresh or, occasionally, lightly steamed fruit. Choose fish or white meat such as poultry (chicken breast without the skin) rather than red meat such as beef or pork. Drink six large glasses of filtered water daily, and experiment with the many blends of herb teas or grain coffee substitutes that are currently available until you find a range of flavors you enjoy.

Guard against constipation by eating regular and plentiful quantities of dietary fiber from whole grains, pulses, and wholemeal bread. Keep dietary fat to a minimum (butter, eggs, cheeses, and margarines) as an additional way of avoiding constipation.

If you are overweight, shedding excess pounds will help a great deal in taking the extra strain off your weight-bearing joints such as hips, knees, and ankles.

Food supplements that may be helpful in relieving joint problems include vitamins that support the detoxifying activities of the body, such as vitamins C and B complex, cod liver oil, and extract of green-lipped mussel.

EXERCISE
Keep mobile in order to prevent your joints from seizing up. By exercising regularly from our middle years onward, we can do a great deal to protect our joints, keeping them as free and flexible as possible. Choose exercise that appeals to you and fits

Typical Features	General Symptoms
Joint pains that are relieved by movement	"Rusty gate" syndrome: stiff, painful joints that are very painful when sitting still or lying down. Once limbered up, joints become much more comfortable. Depressed with pains in bed at night.
Joint pains that are painful for slightest movement	Painful, inflamed joints that respond well to a night's rest. Stitching pains with swollen, pale pink swelling around the affected joint. General state of toxicity with joint pains, including constipation and headaches. Irritable and antisocial with pain.
Hot, stiff, painful joints that are eased by cool bathing	Joint pains that start in the feet and move upward. Pains affect joints on opposite sides of the body. Joints become mis-shapen in feet and hands and are very sensitive to pressure.
Weak, painful knee joints that "give out" when moving	Low back pain accompanies discomfort in joints. Stiff, painful joints that are much worse for exposure to damp, cold conditions. Unsteady from weak feeling in weight-bearing joints.
Swollen, stinging joints that are aggravated by warmth	Puffy swelling around painful joints that feel immediately relieved by cool bathing. General state of fluid retention may accompany joint problems with taut feeling in affected areas. Very irritable and fidgety with pain.
Tearing, raw pains that develop slowly	Stiffness and pain in joints with severe discomfort in the knee joint. Cracking in knee joint when getting up from sitting position or when walking. "Restless legs" at night with difficulty finding a comfortable position.
Painful joints after eating too many rich or fatty foods	Weak, swollen joints that are much better for being moved. Heavy, bruised feeling in legs that are restless and achy at night. Shifting, changeable pains that move from joint to joint. Very weepy and depressed with pains.

Better for	Worse from	Remedy
Warm bath or shower Continued motion Heat applied to painful areas Dry, warm conditions	Cold and damp Overexertion At night Getting up from sitting position Standing	Rhus tox.
Keeping as still as possible Firm pressure Lying on the painful area	Slightest movement Physical effort Warmth	Bryonia
Cold bathing Contact with cool air Cold locally applied	Becoming warm in bed Pressure Movement Damp weather Alcohol	Ledum
Gentle exercise indoors Dry warmth	Resting Cold, damp weather Pressure Lying on painful joint	Ruta
Cool bathing Contact with cool air Movement	Warm bathing Heat locally applied Keeping still Lying down Damp Touch	Apis
Warm, humid weather Being warm in bed	Exposure to dry, cold winds Dry weather After bathing Coffee	Causticum
Cool bathing Gentle exercise in the open air Firm pressure Weeping Sympathy	Becoming heated At night Heavy bedcovers Keeping still or lying down Initial movement	Pulsatilla

your daily routine with the minimum amount of fuss. Excellent methods include walking, swimming, and cycling. General activities to be avoided include any exercise involving repetitive pounding, jarring movements such as jogging or running on hard surfaces.

Attending a regular yoga class can be very beneficial. Yoga classes are noncompetitive, and a good teacher will never encourage anyone to attempt a posture that is beyond their physical capacity. However, well-executed yoga postures are challenging and enable us to develop stamina, strength, and flexibility. Always inform your yoga teacher if you suffer from joint problems: he or she can ensure that you do not attempt any inappropriate postures, which may put undue strain on already damaged joints.

VARICOSE VEINS

Problems with varicose veins are often an inherited condition or develop during pregnancy due to the extra strain put on the circulatory system at this time. Veins are different from arteries because they do not have such elastic walls and do not benefit as much from the vigorous pumping motion of the heart. As a result, the upward movement of blood through the major veins in the lower limbs is totally dependant on the muscular contractions of the legs and the effective working of a system of valves within the veins, which prevents the backflow of blood.

Unfortunately, these valves can become less efficient over time, creating greater pressure on the veins, resulting in the characteristic knobbly or distended appearance of varicose veins. The problems associated with varicose veins can vary from mild irritation or discomfort to severe pain and ulceration of the skin surrounding the affected vein or veins.

Homeopathic Help

If your symptoms are severe, or if you suffer from general circulatory problems, it is advisable to seek treatment from a homeopathic practitioner to achieve the most positive outcome.

However, if your symptoms are very mild, you may find an occasional dose of the appropriately selected remedy may help a great deal with the general discomfort, aching, or itching of your condition. As always, it is best to combine homeopathic prescribing with the general advice on self-help given below.

Practical Self-Help

REST
Avoid standing for any length of time. Also make sure you rest as often as possible with your feet up.

CLOTHING
If you suspect you have a tendency toward varicose veins, avoid wearing hold-up stockings or any other items of clothing that apply pressure to the thighs or hips. Use support stockings or tights and avoid crossing your legs when sitting.

WEIGHT
Carrying excess weight can compound the problems of varicose veins. See the advice given in the section "Weight Gain" in chapter 4 (p. 51).

EXERCISE
Regular aerobic exercise is essential if you suffer from circulatory problems such as varicose veins. Choose rhythmic movement that avoids jarring or jolting, such as brisk walking or cycling.

Typical Features	General Symptoms
Varicose veins with easy bruising	Very sensitive to pain with stiffness and aching in the legs. Discomfort is worse in bed: tosses and turns constantly in an effort to get comfortable. Feet may be swollen and legs feel bruised.
Left-sided varicose veins	Problems may be restricted to the left leg, or may spread from left to right. Bursting, pounding pains in legs that are worse for contact with heat. Feels better for activities that stimulate the circulation such as walking.
Right-sided varicose veins with a tendency to ulceration	Shifting, changeable pains with heavy sensations in legs. Symptoms may be restricted to right leg, or worse on that side. Veins become congested during pregnancy. Poor circulation in hands and feet. Weepy and in need of sympathy when in pain.
Bruised feeling in legs with prickling pains in veins	One of the main remedies to consider for varicose veins, if individualizing characteristics are difficult to spot. Intense, sore pains: sensation of blood being forced through veins. Poor circulation with tendency to chilblains.
Burning, itching varicose veins with a tendency to ulcerate	Varicose veins affect legs, arms, and vulva. Internal burning sensations that are relieved by exposure to cool, fresh air. Pulsating pains in legs with cramps in calves at night.
Burning pains in veins that are much better for warmth	Very restless with pains, especially at night. Always cold because of poor circulation. Feeling as though waves of burning, or ice-cold blood are coursing through veins.

Better for	Worse from	Remedy
Lying with head lower than the body	Touch Movement Alcohol Damp, cold conditions	Arnica
Cool air Coolness, applied locally to the painful area Onset of a period pain	Warmth Keeping still After a night's rest Before a period Tight clothing	Lachesis
Cool air Cool bathing Gentle exercise in the open air Pressure, or lying on painful side Uncovering	Becoming too hot Heavy clothes or bedcovers Lying or sitting still Becoming chilled or damp	Pulsatilla
Night	Touch Movement During the day In open air	Hamamelis
Fresh, cool air Being fanned After sleep	Warmth Stuffy rooms Humidity Movement Chill	Carbo veg.
Warm surroundings Heat applied to painful part Resting in a warm bed Company	Becoming chilled or damp Cold applied locally At night Worrying about health	Arsenicum album

DIET

If you are constipated, rectify the problem by including more fiber in your diet from fresh fruit, vegetables, pulses, and whole grains. Also ensure that you drink a minimum of five large glasses of filtered water daily. Avoid overly processed or refined foods and items that contain a large amount of fat, especially eggs and dairy foods such as full-fat cheese and cream.

Consider supplementing your diet with vitamins and other nutrients that have a reputation for improving circulation. These include vitamin B_3 (part of the B vitamin complex), vitamin C, and vitamin E. Rutin has a reputation for reducing the misery of varicose veins by strengthening the walls of the veins. It can be taken in supplement form or can be introduced into the diet in the form of buckwheat.

TOPICAL APPLICATIONS

If your skin has a tendency to ulcerate, apply Calendula cream to the affected area at the first sign of a problem. Calendula is immensely soothing, and acts as an effective antiseptic, encouraging the skin to heal rapidly. Although Arnica may be taken internally if indicated for varicose veins, never apply Arnica cream to broken skin: always choose Calendula or Hypercal™ (a combination of Hypericum and Calendula) instead.

6

Hormone Replacement Therapy:
The Controversy

Few methods of medical treatment have attracted the media coverage that hormone replacement therapy (HRT) has over the past few years. Many female celebrities have sung its praises, and discussions about menopause on television and in the press are not complete without an opinion being voiced about HRT.

Since we are most likely to be offered HRT by our GPs as the treatment of choice, if we experience unpleasant symptoms as we approach menopause, it is essential that we understand the implications of accepting or opting out of treatment by HRT.

THE ORTHODOX MEDICAL VIEW

Many conventional doctors regard menopausal women as experiencing a hormone deficiency, which can be supplemented by providing extra estrogen in the form of HRT. Treatment may be given in the form of pills, patches (applied to the skin), implants (surgically inserted beneath the skin), or in cream or gel form (applied to areas that are thinning, or becoming painful, such as the wall of the vagina).

Symptoms that may respond well to treatment with HRT include:

- hot flashes;
- night sweats;
- painful and weakened joints as a result of osteoporosis (brittle bones);
- dryness or inflammation of the vaginal wall;
- depression;
- poor memory and lack of concentration;
- fatigue and low energy levels;
- insomnia or poor quality sleep;
- diminished libido;
- dry skin or poor skin tone.

Conventional doctors also stress that the estrogen component of HRT protects the heart and circulatory system, reducing the risks of heart attacks or strokes. Estrogen is also thought to protect the quality of our bones, making them less susceptible to easy fracture and other problems of osteoporosis.

The Alternative Viewpoint

Although the claims of the proponents of HRT are very attractive and many women feel at ease with taking it, there are certain problems associated with its use that need to be taken into consideration. We do not know yet what the long-term effects of HRT may be, and we may not have a full picture of the possible side effects for some time to come. However, we already know that there are certain drawbacks or risks associated with the use of HRT. These include the following:

- an increased possibility of developing cancer of the breast or endometrium (lining of the womb);
- raised blood pressure;

- fibroids;
- increased chance of developing gallstones;
- irregular bleeding;
- weight gain;
- mood swings;
- fluid retention;
- acne or greasy skin.

Many women, especially if they are elderly, find it unacceptable to go back to having a monthly period once they have gone through menopause. It is the progesterone component of HRT that causes monthly bleeding. Without it, the endometrium (lining of the womb) would build up each month rather than being shed, with the possible attendant risk of cancer developing in the womb.

The progesterone element of HRT may also aggravate symptoms that resemble premenstrual syndrome (PMS). These include: mood swings, anxiety, irritability, breast tenderness, sleep problems, acne, and fluid retention. However, progesterone is seen as being a necessary ingredient, because of the increased risk of developing uterine cancer that is associated with an estrogen–only formulation.

There are certain contraindications to the use of HRT, which a GP would consider when deciding whether to prescibe the treatment. These include the following conditions:

- a history of breast or endometrial cancer;
- liver disease.

Additional conditions to be taken into consideration include:

- endometriosis;
- circulatory problems or heart disease;
- chest problems related to heavy smoking.

OSTEOPOROSIS

Additional questions have been raised about the treatment of osteoporosis by HRT. Enthusiasts for HRT point out that it will protect against the loss of bone density that occurs after menopause. However, it cannot repair damage that may have been done before HRT is taken, and it will only protect bone density while treatment is taking place. In other words, it does not have a long-term protective effect, and protracted drug therapy is needed to preserve bone strength. This is a major drawback for those of us who are uneasy about taking hormone treatment for an indefinite period.

It is also important to remember that we can take a variety of positive steps to protect and preserve the quality of our bones as we go through menopause. These include the following.

CALCIUM INTAKE
We should ensure that we have an adequate supply of calcium in our diets. The recommended daily amount (RDA) for women who are not taking HRT is 1,500 mg of calcium per day at the age of forty, which can be reduced gradually to 1,200 mg at the age of sixty and over. For women who are taking HRT the RDA is 1,000 mg. Apart from dairy foods, we can also obtain calcium from green leafy vegetables, seeds, nuts, fish (those eaten with bones, such as sardines), and wholemeal bread. For those of us who are concerned about the fat content in dairy products, it is interesting to note that semiskimmed and skimmed milk have a higher calcium content than full-fat milk.

LOOKING AHEAD
We must be aware of the need to look after our bones well before menopause begins. By the age of thirty-five, we have reached our peak bone mass. At this stage, the strength and quality of our bones will determine whether we are likely to be at risk of devel-

oping osteoporosis after menopause. If we have teenage daughters, therefore, we need to be sure that they are getting adequate quantities of calcium in their diet. This can be particularly difficult, since many girls tend to crash diet at this time, often with disastrous results for their bone density in the future. It is never too late to begin looking at your calcium intake, but the sooner you do so the better.

OTHER NUTRIENTS

For the maximum amount of calcium to be absorbed by our bodies, we need to ensure that we are taking adequate supplies of vitamin D and magnesium. Vitamin D is essential for regulating the amount of calcium that is absorbed by our bodies and the ratio that is filtered out through our kidneys. We can obtain vitamin D by exposing our skin to sunlight and from eating oily fish (mackerel, herrings, salmon, or sardines), egg yolk, and fortified products such as milk or margarines. Magnesium can be obtained from soybeans, nuts, brown rice, seafood, wholemeal bread, and green leafy vegetables.

ESTROGEN

The hormone estrogen is also essential for the maximum utilization of calcium. Although levels of estrogen drop dramatically as we go through menopause, we should be aware that regular exercise stimulates small amounts of estrogen secretion. Other factors that diminish estrogen production include: having a very low body weight, smoking, and drinking regular or large amounts of alcohol and strong coffee.

EXERCISE

Become as physically active as possible. The best form of movement for protecting the strength and quality of our bones is any weight-bearing exercise. This includes brisk walking, jogging, cycling, and low-impact aerobics. If you already experience pain or suspect a weakness in some of your joints, it is best to avoid jogging, because the repetitive jarring movements may aggravate any existing weaknesses. Alternate other exercises with weight-bearing movement such as swimming, yoga, and stretching.

FLUIDS
Drink moderate amounts of alcohol, well within your daily limit of one to two units, and ensure that you have alcohol-free weeks or months. Drink as much mineral or filtered water as possible, and remember that caffeinated drinks increase the leaching of calcium from our bones.

OTHER CONVENTIONAL MEDICATION

Although HRT is most likely to be prescribed for menopausal problems, there are other orthodox drugs that may be used. These include:

- tranquilizers;
- antidepressants;
- beta-blockers;
- drug therapy for osteoporosis of the spine;
- clonidine.

Tranquilizers

Many of us have become uneasy about the routine prescription of tranquilizers, because of concerns about the much-publicized problems of addiction or dependency. While tranquilizers may dull the trauma of anxiety in the short run, they often cease to be helpful after prolonged use, especially if the original problems that gave rise to the anxiety have not been resolved. They also can lead to distressing side effects when withdrawn after extended use. Withdrawal from tranquilizers should be a slow and gentle process, reducing the dose by half a tablet every five days.

For information on homeopathic and self-help treatments that can be used as an alternative to tranquilizers, see the section "Anxiety" in chapter 3 (p. 23).

Antidepressants

Antidepressants may be prescribed for depressive feelings that arise during menopause. It has been suggested that antidepressants are not addictive. However, there are common side effects, which may include:

- dry mouth;
- blurred vision;
- drowsiness;
- lowered libido;
- impaired urine function;
- constipation.

Like tranquilizers, antidepressants should never be withdrawn abruptly, but should be reduced very gradually under professional supervision.

For information on homeopathic and self-help treatments that can be used as an alternative to antidepressants, see the section "Depression" in chapter 3 (p. 35).

Beta-blockers

Although mainly used to control symptoms of high blood pressure or migraine, beta-blockers such as Propranalol may be prescribed for the treatment of hot flashes. Side effects may include:

- digestive problems;
- slow pulse;
- peripheral circulatory problems, such as chilblains;
- particular problems for diabetics or asthmatics.

For information on homeopathic and self-help treatments for hot flashes, see the section "Hot Flashes and Night Sweats" in chapter 5 (p. 72).

Drug Therapy for Osteoporosis of the Spine

Etidronate is a drug that encourages bone-building cells to work more effectively, and slows down the action of cells that break down bone. It is therefore used to treat osteoporosis of the spine. Side effects may include:

- nausea;
- diarrhea;
- increased aching in bones and joints.

For information on homeopathic and self-help methods for the treatment and prevention of osteoporosis, see the section "Osteoporosis" in chapter 4 (p. 61).

Clonidine

This is a drug that has been used in the treatment of migraines and high blood pressure, and which may reduce the frequency of hot flashes. Side effects include:

- dizziness;
- dry mouth;
- nausea;

- skin rashes;
- drowsiness.

For information on homeopathic and self-help treatments for hot flashes, see the section "Hot Flashes and Night Sweats" in chapter 5 (p. 72).

7

~

Checklist of Homeopathic Remedies

The information given below will be very helpful if you are having difficulties in selecting an appropriate homeopathic remedy from the tables given in chapters 3, 4, and 5. Before consulting this section, read the practical information given in chapter 2.

ACONITE

Key Features

Aconite is indicated in the following circumstances.

- Crises arise rapidly, violently, and unexpectedly—for example, symptoms develop after a shock or trauma, such as witnessing an accident or hearing distressing news.
- Symptoms develop as a result of exposure to chill or very cold winds.
- There is a terrible physical and mental restlessness and a sense of panic or terror.
- Intolerance of pain accompanies most symptoms.
- The remedy is required in the early stage of illness and tends to be fast-acting.

Emotions

Aconite may be required where the patient:

- has an overwhelming sense of panic and a conviction that death is near, which may be so strong that the time of death is predicted;
- is frantic and very easily startled with panic;
- is afraid of the dark, crowded places, and of going out;
- is beside herself with impatience and demands that something must be done at once;
- is afraid of being approached or touched;
- has palpitations with anxiety or panic.

Specific Symptoms

Aconite is indicated when the following symptoms occur.

HOT FLASHES
- Hot flashes come on rapidly and violently.
- Panic and anxiety precede or accompany the flashes.
- The head and face are burning hot, while the rest of the body feels cold and clammy.

SLEEP
- Problems emerge or get much worse at night.
- There is very restless insomnia.

HEADACHE
- There is a sudden onset of violent headache with dizziness.
- Head pains or facial neuralgia may follow a shock or fright.
- The head feels burning hot with severe headache.
- Headaches are made worse by moving, talking, sitting up, or drinking.

CYSTITIS AND KIDNEY PROBLEMS

- There is a sudden, violent onset of cutting, sharp pains, with scanty amounts of urine being passed.
- Urine may be blood-streaked.
- Problems may follow shock or emotional trauma.

JOINTS AND MUSCLES

- The patient is oversensitive to pain in the joints and may cry out when walking.
- Joint pains cause weakness in the hips and knees.
- Arms and legs feel numb, heavy, or bruised.

Symptoms are better

- after a sound sleep;
- when perspiring;
- in the fresh air.

Symptoms are worse

- from exposure to cold winds;
- after emotional trauma or shock;
- in extreme temperatures;
- from alcohol;
- at night.

AGNUS CASTUS

Key Features

Agnus castus is indicated in the following circumstances.

- Libido and sex drive are low as a result of a general lowering of energy and vitality.
- There is a state of extreme indifference and apathy.
- Although the body feels warm to the touch, there is an inner sensation of chilliness or sensations of coldness alternate with flashes of heat.
- There are sensations of heaviness because of weak or poorly toned muscles.
- Bruise-type pain can occur anywhere in the body.

Emotions

Agnus castus may be required where the patient:

- is depressed and weary from overall exhaustion;
- is forgetful and inclined to lose her train of thought and the thread of a conversation;
- has a strong fixation about disease and a fear of death, with a conviction that she is going to die soon;
- experiences rapid mood swings, shifting from depression to euphoria very abruptly;
- alternates between confidence and complete lack of self-esteem;
- has no pleasure or enjoyment from life, with a conviction that the best years have gone and that there is nothing to look forward to.

Specific Symptoms

Agnus castus is indicated for the following symptoms.

HEADACHE
- Pains in the head are much worse with movement, especially of the eyes. Reading also makes the headache worse.

- Head pains lodge on the top of the head, above the right eye, or in the right temple.

APPETITE AND DIGESTION
- Nausea and queasiness are much worse while standing.
- Hunger is not satisfied by eating.
- Colicky pains are worse for pressure on the abdomen from sitting.
- There are dragging sensations in the rectum, with difficulty passing stools.

CYSTITIS AND KIDNEY PROBLEMS
- There is a frequent need to pass a large quantity of dark-colored urine, with distressing discomfort after urination.
- There is total aversion to sexual activity with generalized exhaustion or lack of interest.
- Heavy, extended periods last for two weeks.
- Prolapse occurs with weak, drooping sensations.

JOINTS AND MUSCLES
- Joints are easily dislocated, or pains may date from old strains and sprains that have never healed properly.
- Joints lack flexibility.

Symptoms are better

- after resting;
- when keeping as still as possible.

Symptoms are worse

- with movement;
- after exertion.

ANACARDIUM

Key Features

Anacardium is indicated in the following circumstances.

- Severe mood swings are related to fluctuations in hormonal levels: for example, before a period or at menopause.
- The patient is constantly fidgety, restless, or exhausted.
- There is a general sense of pressure or a constriction that may occur anywhere in the body and that may feel like a lump, plug, or hoop.

Emotions

Anacardium may be required where the patient:

- has a characteristic sense of being two people, or having two opposing wills pulling in opposite directions;
- feels obliged to do things against her will or natural inclination;
- has the sensation that her mind and body are separate, making everything seem unreal or in a dream;
- has fixed ideas and may be convinced that someone is watching or following her;
- is depressed and despondent.

Other symptoms

Anacardium is indicated when the following symptoms occur.

HOT FLASHES
- Although generally very chilly, evening or night sweats occur. These affect the head, back, and belly.

SLEEP

- The patient wakes unrefreshed after disturbing dreams of fire, dead bodies, or heights.

HEADACHE

- General exhaustion leads to headaches with dizziness and confusion.
- Head pains are made worse by movement and bending the head backward. Eating improves the situation.

APPETITE AND DIGESTION

- Nausea occurs on waking.
- The patient must eat regularly to keep hunger pangs at bay.
- Stomach pains are relieved by warm food and aggravated by cold drinks.
- There is a nasty taste in the mouth when not eating.
- Constipation occurs, with a "plugged" sensation.

CYSTITIS AND KIDNEY PROBLEMS

- A constant urge to urinate is especially bad at night.

GYNECOLOGICAL PROBLEMS

- Vaginal discharge occurs, with itching or burning around the entrance to the vagina.
- Periods are scanty and frequent, or there is "spotting" between periods.

JOINTS AND MUSCLES

- When keeping still, parts of the body go quickly to sleep.
- Knees give out on walking: they feel constricted, as though they have a tight bandage around them.
- There are frequent bouts of pain and cramp, which are especially bad at night or when walking.

Symptoms are better

- after eating;
- in the evenings;
- after resting.

Symptoms are worse

- on an empty stomach;
- with exposure to cold and drafts;
- after physical effort;
- in the mornings.

APIS

Key Features

Apis is indicated in the following circumstances.

- Allergic reactions cause symptoms that affect the skin, eyes, chest, or throat.
- Characteristic swellings are puffy, pink, and waterlogged, and "pit" on pressure (a dimple is left in the swelling after applying pressure).
- Pains are severe and sting or burn. They are much worse for exposure to warmth, and much better for contact with cold.

Emotions

Apis may be required where the patient:

- develops symptoms after an emotional shock or upset;
- is very fidgety, restless, and irritable;

- is afraid of having a stroke;
- is emotionally volatile and unstable;
- is hypersensitive and tearful;
- wants attention and company but rejects affection.

Other symptoms

Apis is indicated when the following symptoms occur.

HOT FLASHES
- The head and face are hot and sweaty, and the patient craves cool air.
- She tosses and turns at night in search of a cool place in the bed, and throws off the bedcovers to cool down.

HEADACHE
- Dizziness accompanies a headache, which is better for moving about and worse for lying down or shutting the eyes.
- Throbbing, burning pains occur, which are worse in a warm room.
- There is a fuzzy or thick feeling in the head that feels better with pressure.

CYSTITIS AND KIDNEY PROBLEMS
- Burning, scanty, scalding urine has to be passed frequently.
- There is little or no thirst with kidney problems.
- Fluid retention occurs with kidney disorders, leading to a watery, puffy swelling around the eyes.
- Pains are relieved by contact with anything cool.

GYNECOLOGICAL PROBLEMS
- Pain is felt in the ovary and is usually worse on the right side.

- There are burning and stinging pains in the pelvic region.

JOINTS AND MUSCLES
- There are burning, stinging pains in the joints, which feel better when kept cool.
- Painful joints look swollen, puffy, rosy-pink, shiny, and taut.
- Although the feet may feel cold, the toes look red and inflamed.
- Hands and feet are swollen.

Symptoms are better

- with cold in any form;
- with movement;
- in the fresh open air;
- after uncovering.

Symptoms are worse

- with heat in any form;
- when keeping still;
- in stuffy rooms;
- after a warm bath;
- at night;
- after sleep;
- with touch or pressure.

ARGENTUM NITRICUM (ARG. NIT.)

Key Features

Arg. nit. is one of the main anxiety remedies, and is indicated in the following circumstances.

- The anxiety is linked to anticipation of a coming stressful event.
- Digestive disturbances, such as flatulence and diarrhea, are set off by severe anxiety.
- There is a marked craving for sweets or salt, which aggravate the general condition.
- Pains are characteristically constricting or squeezing in nature.

Emotions

Arg. nit. may be required where the patient:

- has constant feelings of agitation, restlessness, and anxiety about what may happen;
- is afraid when anticipating a coming event or anxious about crowded places, heights, closed-in spaces, or bridges;
- is constantly on the move as a way of coping with agitation: as soon as one job is done she has to move on to the next.

Specific Symptoms

Arg. nit. is indicated when the following symptoms occur.

HOT FLASHES
- Anxiety brings on sudden, copious sweats.

SLEEP
- The patient cannot get comfortable in bed because of feeling too cold when lightly covered and too hot with extra bedcovers.
- Anxiety about a coming event causes severe insomnia.
- She feels exhausted and aching all over on waking.

HEADACHE
- The head feels enlarged when painful; discomfort is relieved by tight pressure.
- Throbbing pains are made worse by warmth and relieved by cool.

APPETITE AND DIGESTION
- A sick feeling is relieved by eating.
- The patient feels nauseated and distended soon after eating; belching or passing wind do not help.
- Nervous diarrhea is aggravated by eating sweet things.

CYSTITIS AND KIDNEY PROBLEMS
- Nervous upsets may lead to pain on passing scanty urine, with scalding sensations during and after urination.
- Urine may contain traces of blood.

GYNECOLOGICAL PROBLEMS
- Periods are very painful, with an intermittent yellow discharge.
- There is inflammation and discomfort around the entrance to the vagina, with sharp, sticking pains.

JOINTS AND MUSCLES
- Pains mainly affect the small joints in the hands and feet.
- Back pain is especially bad when sitting or rising from a sitting position. It is relieved by walking or standing.

Symptoms are better

- in the fresh air;
- when wearing light clothing;
- with firm pressure.

Symptoms are worse

- with warmth;
- in stuffy rooms;
- after eating sugary foods;
- at night;
- during emotional strain;
- on waking.

ARNICA

Key Features

Arnica is the first remedy to think of in any accident, fall, shock, bruising, or muscular overexertion. Because of its effectiveness as a trauma remedy, it is often the first remedy bought by newcomers to homeopathy. It is indicated in the following circumstances.

- Arnica is used for dealing with both the physical and emotional reactions to shock and for speeding overall recovery.
- Pains are generally bruised, aching, and oversensitive to touch.
- There is a tendency to bruise easily.

Emotions

Arnica may be required where the patient:

- pushes everyone away, insisting that there is nothing wrong;
- has a terrible fear and anxiety about being approached because of sensitivity to pain;

- is withdrawn and morose and wants to be left alone in peace;
- is forgetful and has difficulty in concentrating;
- is irritable and easily disturbed.

Specific Symptoms

Arnica is indicated when the following symptoms occur.

HOT FLASHES
- Flashes of heat may affect the upper half of the body, while the lower half remains cool.
- Severe palpitations occur with hot flashes.

SLEEP
- The patient is sleepless because of aching or feeling bruised all over.
- She wakes between 2:00 and 3:00 A.M., often from disturbed dreams or nightmares.
- She tosses and turns because the bed feels too hard to sleep on.

HEADACHE
- A sick headache is worse on closing the eyes.
- The headache is one-sided, with a sharp pain, as though a nail were being pushed into the skull.

APPETITE AND DIGESTION
- The patient is excessively thirsty for cold drinks, or in contrast, has no thirst at all.
- She craves sour condiments such as vinegar or alcohol.
- She is nauseated by the idea of eating.

CYSTITIS AND KIDNEY PROBLEMS
- There is a constant desire to urinate, with great difficulty in starting the flow.

- Urination is difficult after too much exercise.
- Urine may contain bloody deposits.

JOINTS AND MUSCLES
- There are heavy, aching sensations in the arms and legs, with exhaustion and weariness.
- Too much physical exercise and muscle strain give rise to general bruised, sore sensations.
- Hands are swollen or feet feel sore and bruised.
- All pains are worse from exposure to cold and damp.

Symptoms are better

- when lying with the head lower than the body.

Symptoms are worse

- from overexposure to hot, sunny conditions;
- when it's cold and damp;
- with excessive amounts of exercise;
- on being approached or touched;
- from drinking alcohol.

ARSENICUM ALBUM

Key Features

Arsenicum album is indicated in the following circumstances.

- There is extreme anxiety and physical and mental restlessness.
- Marked mental and physical tiredness may come on very rapidly.

- All symptoms get much worse with the onset of night and in the dark.
- There is extreme chilliness with a strong aversion to any contact with cold.
- Burning pains are relieved by warmth.
- Nausea, vomiting, and diarrhea occur together.

Emotions

Arsenicum album may be required where the patient:

- is overwhelmingly restless and anxious, pacing around the room in an effort to keep calm;
- has specific fears about illness, being alone, darkness, and dying;
- has anxiety leading to obsessional behavior, such as needing to organize the family and get on with daily chores, even when too tired to do so;
- becomes unreasonably concerned about hygiene and contamination from germs, because of fear of food poisoning;
- is oversensitive to noise, smells, and pain;
- becomes depressed and despondent when ill, to the point of feeling that very little can be done;
- is fastidious about appearance, surroundings, and work;
- has high standards and is therefore critical of others or of her own achievements.

Specific Symptoms

Arsenicum album is indicated when the following symptoms occur.

HOT FLASHES
- Although the patient is chilly by nature, flashes of burning heat sweep through the body from head to toe.

SLEEP

- The patient wakes at around 1:00 A.M., sweating and anxious.
- She suffers from insomnia and restlessness and is compelled to get up in the early hours and make a cup of tea.

HEADACHE

- Migraine headaches occur with severe anxiety, restlessness, nausea, and vomiting.
- Headaches feel worse with bright light, noise, and movement.
- The head is the only part of the body that feels better for contact with cool air or cool applications.
- Pains are throbbing and burning, and may be brought on by anxiety, overexcitement, or becoming overheated.

APPETITE AND DIGESTION

- Acidity and burning pains in the stomach are relieved by sips of warm drinks and made worse by cool drinks.
- Although the stomach is very sensitive to touch, it feels soothed by warm applications.

CYSTITIS AND KIDNEY PROBLEMS

- Cystitis causes great distress and anxiety with burning pains when urinating.
- Kidney problems give rise to chilliness, nausea, restlessness, and prostration.
- Fluid retention results from kidney disorders and causes puffiness around the eyes.

GYNECOLOGICAL PROBLEMS

- Period pains are severe and there is vomiting, diarrhea, restlessness, and anxiety.

- There is marked irritation of the vagina with burning, watery discharge, and sensitivity to touch.

JOINTS AND MUSCLES
- Pain and discomfort in legs at night leads to restlessness and insomnia.
- Backache between the shoulder blades is relieved by resting and lying down.

Symptoms are better

- in warm surroundings;
- with warm applications;
- when taking sips of warm drinks;
- with movement;
- when sitting propped up in bed;
- after sweating.

Symptoms are worse

- when alone;
- at night;
- with chill;
- when taking cold food and drinks;
- from drinking alcohol.

BELLADONNA

Key Features

Situations that respond well to Belladonna tend to flare up rapidly, violently, and with very little warning. It is indicated in the following circumstances.

- The skin is characteristically bright red, dry, and burning hot to the touch.
- All senses are painfully overacute and oversensitive, so touch, light, and noise cannot be tolerated.
- There is extreme irritability and restlessness, especially in those who are normally placid and mild.
- Pains are throbbing, pounding, and pulsating.

Emotions

Belladonna may be required where the patient:

- is agitated and restless, but not terrorstricken or fearful (where Aconite would be indicated);
- is in a semidelirious state with high fever;
- speaks very quickly while seeming in a world of her own;
- is easily overexcited and startled.

Other Symptoms

Belladonna is indicated when the following symptoms occur.

HOT FLASHES
- Circulation is very uneven, with a tendency to feel boiling hot.
- Head is hot and burning while hands and feet are icy cold.
- Bright red flush rapidly spreads over the skin, making it hot, dry, and burning.

SLEEP
- Sleep is disturbed and restless.
- The patient wakes with a start as she is about to fall asleep.
- She twitches and jerks in her sleep or grinds her teeth.

Checklist of Homeopathic Remedies

HEADACHE

- Throbbing, pounding pains are worse for bright lights, noises, or movement.
- Pains are often right-sided and accompanied by dizziness, which is worse when turning over in bed.

APPETITE AND DIGESTION

- Although thirsty for acidic drinks such as lemonade, drinking may be difficult because of pain or swelling in the throat.
- Taste becomes oversensitive or acute.
- There are colicky, cramping pains in the stomach and a desire to bend backward in order to feel comfortable.

CYSTITIS AND KIDNEY PROBLEMS

- Extremely severe bladder problems occur, with cutting, burning pains, and a constant desire to urinate.
- Cramping, constricting pains are very distressing after urination.
- Urine is dark, cloudy, and blood-streaked.
- Stress incontinence occurs while standing or walking.

GYNECOLOGICAL PROBLEMS

- Periods are flooding, with a bright red, clotted flow.
- Menstrual flow feels hot and is accompanied by a severe bearing-down sensation.
- Prolapse occurs, with a sensation that everything is about to fall out of the pelvic cavity.
- Periods are irregular or too early, with extreme cramping, throbbing pains.

JOINTS AND MUSCLES

- Joint problems cause extreme restlessness and a need to keep constantly moving.

- Joints look bright red, swollen, and hot. They are worse for exposure to cold and better for warm applications and keeping still.
- A stiff, painful neck may follow exposure to cold drafts, or becoming damp.

Symptoms are better

- with warmth;
- with peace and quiet;
- after resting;
- when bending the head backward;
- with wrapping up warmly.

Symptoms are worse

- when lying on the painful area;
- with movement of any kind;
- with jarring;
- in bright light;
- with noise;
- with exposure to cold drafts;

BRYONIA

Key Features

Bryonia is indicated in the following circumstances.

- The skin is dry and red and there is intolerance of heat and warmth.

- Because of general picture of dryness, stubborn constipation occurs with resulting toxic symptoms of headache and joint pains.
- Skin and mucous membranes are very dry and sensitive, giving rise to problems such as painful dryness and sensitivity of the vagina.
- All symptoms are made much worse by movement of any kind and relieved by firm pressure.
- Symptoms develop slowly and insidiously and may be sparked off by exposure to abrupt change of temperature, cold or east winds, or by anger, resentment, or fright.

Emotions

Bryonia may be required where the patient:

- is irritable and bad-tempered with illness, with an overwhelming desire to be left alone in peace;
- avoids making any kind of effort, including making conversation;
- is depressed and discontented, with an overwhelming feeling of not knowing what she wants;
- is anxious about work and domestic affairs;
- is angry and abusive if crossed or contradicted in anything.

Specific Symptoms

Bryonia is indicated when the following symptoms occur.

SLEEP
- The patient feels drowsy during the day but unable to sleep soundly at night.
- She may walk in her sleep or be subject to nightmares.

HEADACHE

- On waking, a terrible headache lodges across the eyes or at the back of the head.
- Pains are bursting and throbbing and may be located on the right side of the head.
- Eating, bending forward, and the slightest movement make the pain worse.
- A dull, persistent headache accompanies stubborn constipation.

APPETITE AND DIGESTION

- Indigestion is painful, with a heavy feeling in the stomach.
- Although not in the least hungry, the patient craves large drinks of ice-cold water.
- Warm drinks are soothing.
- Pains in the stomach are sore and tender to touch.
- Constipation is severe, with large, hard, dry stools that are very difficult to pass.

JOINTS AND MUSCLES

- Affected joints look pale red, swollen, and taut.
- Pains are sharp, tearing, and stitching, and very much worse for movement of any kind.
- Although pains are relieved by keeping as still as possible, they may be so severe that the patient cannot keep still, thus causing more pain.
- Walking is difficult because of weak thigh muscles or sore, aching feet.

Symptoms are better

- in cool surroundings and with cool drinks;
- when keeping as still as possible;
- with firm pressure to the affected part;
- from perspiring.

Symptoms are worse

- from warmth and heat in general;
- with movement of any kind;
- when getting up from a sitting position;
- with the first movement after rest.

CALCAREA CARBONICUM (CALC. CARB.)

Key Features

Calc. carb. is indicated in the following circumstances.

- A persistently sluggish or slow metabolism leads to long-term problems with gaining weight.
- All vital processes in the body are slowed down, with resulting poor circulation, constipation, and indigestion.
- The patient is easily exhausted, sweaty, and breathless after very little physical effort.
- She has poor physical stamina and muscle tone, with a tendency to get strains and sprains.
- There are long-term problems with swollen glands and recurrent colds that do not fully clear up.
- Those who require Calc. carb. often experience the unusual symptom of feeling perfectly well when constipated.

Emotions

Calc. carb. may be required where the patient:

- has poor mental and emotional stamina, with a tendency to collapse under pressure;

- lacks confidence and fears being the center of attention or the subject of a joke (this often dates from childhood, when she may have been laughed at or singled out for being overweight, slow, or generally unfit);
- is confused and unable to think clearly under stress;
- becomes uncommunicative or unresponsive as a way of coping with feelings of inadequacy;
- fears being alone, the dark, and anyone noticing her confusion or uncertainty;
- is easily startled and oversensitive to noise;
- becomes depressed and weepy if unable to cope.

Specific Symptoms

Calc. carb. is indicated when the following symptoms occur.

HOT FLASHES
- Although chilly by nature, the patient becomes very quickly hot and bothered if overheated.
- She sweats profusely when exhausted after physical effort or when too hot.
- Night sweats are common as well as drenching sweats from anxiety or overexcitement.
- Hot, burning flashes are quickly followed by a chilled, clammy feeling.

SLEEP
- Problems may date from childhood, with a history of sleepwalking, nightmares, and screaming at night.
- The patient has had long-term difficulties in getting off to sleep, with a tendency to feel anxious at around 2:00 to 4:00 A.M. Alternatively, she may wake at 3:00 A.M. and be unable to get back to sleep.

- Frequent night sweats predominantly affect the head and feet. Feet are pushed out of the bedcovers because they feel burning hot.

HEADACHE
- Headache and dizziness are brought on by exhaustion after physical effort.
- Pain is often right-sided and accompanied by a nauseated, bilious feeling.
- Headaches are made more intense by exposure to bright light, noise, and the effort of talking. They are soothed by warmth and resting in a dark room.

APPETITE AND DIGESTION
- Digestion is slow and inefficient, with resulting nausea and sour belching.
- An empty, faint feeling comes on soon after eating or if a meal is missed.
- Hot food, meat, coffee, and milk are disliked, and may upset the stomach.
- Food cravings may occur for unusual, indigestible things like coal or chalk or for more common foods such as sweets or eggs.
- Constipation is common because of a sluggish digestion, with absolutely no desire to pass a stool.

CYSTITIS AND KIDNEY PROBLEMS
- Cystitis occurs, with sour-smelling, offensive, dark brown urine.

GYNECOLOGICAL PROBLEMS
- There is a right-sided ovarian pain which extends to the thigh.
- Yeast infection with itching and smarting occurs, with a profuse, burning, thick discharge.

- Periods may happen too frequently or too early and go on too long. An irregular pattern may be triggered by too many physical demands or excessive stress.
- Symptoms of PMS may be well established, with a tendency to recurrent breast enlargement and tenderness. These occur before and continue during the period.

JOINTS AND MUSCLES
- There is marked sensitivity to cold and damp, which cause stiffness and pain.
- Strains and sprains occur easily and repeatedly. The ankle joints are especially weak and likely to "twist" easily.
- Joints are hot and swollen and develop gouty or nodular outgrowths.
- Calcium metabolism is poor, leading to poor quality bones or osteoporosis (brittle bones). There may also be a tendency toward curvature of the upper spine as a result of weak muscle tone.
- There are recurrent cramps in calf muscles, especially at night.

Symptoms are better

- with moderate warmth;
- when constipated;
- in dry, warm conditions.

Symptoms are worse

- in cold and damp air;
- with extreme temperature changes;
- when bathing in cold water;
- before and after a period;
- when standing for extended periods of time;
- with physical effort.

CANTHARIS

Key Features

Cantharis is indicated in the following circumstances.

- There is severe internal irritation and burning, with a sensation of external chilliness and shivering.
- Symptoms develop rapidly with very little warning.
- Cantharis has a special affinity for the urinary tract, making it one of the most commonly indicated remedies for the treatment of cystitis.

Emotions

Cantharis may be required where the patient:

- is extremely irritable and oversensitive on mental and physical levels;
- is easily overstimulated or too readily excited;
- becomes drowsy or lethargic when feverish.

Specific Symptoms

Cantharis is indicated when the following symptoms occur.

HEADACHE
- Headaches are violent, with stabbing pains that are eased by walking.
- The headache begins at the back of the head or nape of the neck.

CYSTITIS AND KIDNEY PROBLEMS

- Rapidly developing, burning pains occur before, during, and after urination.
- With cystitis, irritation and discomfort are felt in the bladder and all the way down the urinary tract.
- Burning pains are felt in the kidneys, with a constant desire to urinate.
- Although the genital area is very sensitive and irritated, sexual responsiveness may be heightened.

Symptoms are better

- at night;
- with warmth.

Symptoms are worse

- with touch;
- from drinking coffee;
- with motion.

CARBO VEGETABILIS (CARBO VEG.)

Key Features

Carbo veg. is indicated in the following circumstances.

- There is extreme prostration and faintness, with pallor and a craving for fresh air.
- The circulation is unstable, with problems in efficiently utilizing oxygen intake. This generally leads to constant yawning, stretching, and tiredness.

Emotions

Carbo veg. may be required where the patient:

- is listless and apathetic when ill, with no motivation to become interested in anything;
- has rapid mood changes and may alternate between apathy and marked irritability;
- has mood swings that are worse at night and is anxious in the dark;
- is confused and has a poor memory when depressed.

Specific Symptoms

Carbo veg. is indicated when the following symptoms occur.

HOT FLASHES
- Although the patient is chilly to the core, flashes of heat occur rapidly, and easily.
- Hot flashes are brought on or made worse by drinking wine or eating strongly spiced food.
- Burning heat may be rapidly followed by a severe sense of chill and drenching, clammy sweat.
- Frequent, profuse night sweats interrupt sleep. Clammy perspiration is especially copious on face and limbs.

HEADACHE
- "Morning-after" headaches occur, with throbbing pains or tight sensations across the scalp.
- Severe pains are felt in the temples, with dizziness or a heavy feeling in the head.

APPETITE AND DIGESTION

- Carbo veg. is an excellent remedy for the symptoms of overindulgence, such as nausea, indigestion, or constant belching.
- There are colicky pains in the stomach or abdomen, with an abundance of uncomfortable trapped wind.

JOINTS AND MUSCLES

- The base of the spine is sensitive and painful, and this is much worse when sitting down.
- Bruised, aching sensations in the back, arms, wrists, and small joints of the hands cause constant restlessness and uneasiness.
- Because of poor circulation, parts lain on become numb very quickly.

Symptoms are better

- in the fresh air;
- from being fanned;
- after sleep.

Symptoms are worse

- in stuffy rooms;
- in severely cold conditions;
- with humidity;
- from drinking alcohol;
- from eating;
- with movement.

CAUSTICUM

Key Features

Causticum is indicated in the following circumstances.

- Symptoms develop slowly and insidiously, often as the result of becoming run down by stress or emotional strain.
- Illness is accompanied by increasing exhaustion, with an overwhelming need to rest or lie down.
- The patient feels generally much worse for raw, cold weather with sharp east winds.
- Pains are severe, raw, tearing, or drawing in nature.
- Causticum is appropriate for slowly developing states of paralysis, which may accompany joint problems such as arthritis.

Emotions

Causticum may be required where the patient:

- has been gradually exhausted and worn down from persistent emotional strain, possibly following a period of nursing a sick close relative, loss of sleep, financial strain, or domestic worries;
- becomes readily involved in caring organizations or charities because of an intense capacity to sympathize with others;
- is anxious and lacking in confidence, with a tendency to become easily startled or frightened by the least noise or disturbance;
- has a fear of the dark which may date from childhood and a long-term dread of going to bed in the dark;

- adopts a pose of sarcasm or peevishness as a defense mechanism in an effort to disguise lack of confidence or anxiety;
- displays obsessive behavior, such as repeatedly checking that doors have been locked or electrical appliances switched off as a result of long-term anxiety and insecurity.

Specific Symptoms

Causticum is indicated when the following symptoms occur.

SLEEP
- The patient is totally insomniac at night but drowsy and yawning throughout the day.
- She has "restless legs" at night and cannot get comfortable in bed.
- She starts awake or is unable to get to sleep from disturbing images before the eyes.

HEADACHE
- Headaches are severe and sickly and feel worse in warm surroundings.
- There is a tight feeling in the scalp, which is eased by applying warmth.

DIGESTION AND APPETITE
- There is a raw, burning sensation in the stomach, with acid rising into the throat.
- The abdomen swells after eating, with colicky pains that are better for bending over.
- Hemorrhoids cause raw, burning pains, which are worse when walking or with touch.

BLADDER AND KIDNEY PROBLEMS

- Stress incontinence occurs, with leakage of urine when laughing or becoming excited.
- Leakage of urine is worse at night and improved in summer.
- Slow or difficult flow of urine is eased by drinking cold liquids.
- Itching and irritation occur around the entrance to the urethra.

JOINTS AND MUSCLES

- Joint disorders give rise to raw, tearing pains. The knee joints are especially affected.
- The joints are swollen and stiff and are much worse when rising from a chair.
- Muscle pains develop after overexertion.
- All joint pains are worse during cold, windy weather and improved by contact with damp, warm conditions.

Symptoms are better

- on becoming warm in bed;
- with warmth;
- in damp weather.

Symptoms are worse

- with cold, east winds;
- in dry weather;
- in drafty conditions;
- with abrupt or violent changes of temperature;
- after bathing;
- with movement;
- from drinking coffee;
- at night or on waking.

CHINA (CINCHONA OFFICINALIS)

Key Features

China is indicated in the following circumstances.

- There is severe physical and mental exhaustion, often as a result of a short-term iron-deficiency anemia.
- Pains are cutting, tearing, or sharp.
- Exhaustion follows blood loss, diarrhea, or sweating.
- All the senses are oversensitive, with a dislike of even light touch or the slightest draft of cold air.
- There is a general tendency to fluid retention.
- Symptoms develop after an extended period of physical or emotional strain.

Emotions

China may be required where the patient:

- is touchy and irritable and wants to be left alone;
- is anxious and fearful, especially at night;
- is afraid of insects, dogs, and animals in general;
- is intolerant of and oversensitive to noise because of generally weakened state.

Specific Symptoms

China is indicated when the following symptoms occur.

HOT FLASHES
- Although the patient is generally chilly and shivery, hot flashes of heat occur with hot sweats.
- Night sweats are drenching and frequent.
- Violent thirst often accompanies perspiration and hot flashes.

HEADACHE
- Throbbing headaches are at the sides of the head, and the scalp is very sensitive.
- Pains are much worse with jarring movement, touch, and cold drafts.
- Headaches are improved by firm pressure and warm conditions.

APPETITE AND DIGESTION
- The patient constantly feels full, with little or no appetite.
- There is a cold sensation in the stomach, with a strong desire for stimulants and condiments.
- She feels heavy after eating, with bloating and flatulence.
- Digestive problems are not relieved by passing wind.
- Gall bladder problems or jaundice occur, with digestive uneasiness.
- Diarrhea is watery, offensive, profuse and painless, and is worse at night.

GYNECOLOGICAL PROBLEMS
- There is severe bleeding premenopausally, with marked weariness and exhaustion.
- Menstrual flow is early, very heavy, dark, and mixed with clots.

JOINTS AND MUSCLES
- Legs are weak and trembly when making any kind of physical effort.
- Arms and legs quickly go numb if pressure is applied to them.
- Joint pains are much worse for movement.

Symptoms are better

- after resting;

- with warmth;
- after a hot cup of tea;
- with firm pressure.

Symptoms are worse

- in cold drafts;
- with cold in general;
- with motion;
- with touch;
- at night;
- after eating;
- from eating acid fruits.

CIMICIFUGA RACEMOSA

Key Features

Cimicifuga is indicated in the following circumstances.

- The patient is constantly restless with a frantic need to change position.
- Symptoms shift between physical and emotional levels.
- Symptoms are changeable, and pains tend to flit from place to place.
- Problems are often located on the left side of the body.
- The patient is always chilly and never feels really warm.

Emotions

Cimicifuga may be required where the patient:

- is terribly depressed and gloomy and sighs constantly;

- alternates between depression and euphoria, talkativeness and exhilaration;
- is very suspicious about everyone and everything, including medical treatment;
- fears going insane or dying;
- has health problems following emotional stress or strain.

With Cimicifuga there is a marked tendency for physical problems to improve when emotional symptoms are intense and vice versa.

Specific Symptoms

Cimicifuga is indicated when the following symptoms occur.

HEADACHE
- Pains are severe and much worse for moving or noise or during a period.
- Headaches are eased by cool, fresh air, and pressure.
- Neuralgic pains in the cheek bones improve at night but get worse by the following morning.

APPETITE AND DIGESTION
- Queasiness and vomiting accompany gynecological problems such as painful periods.
- Cramping, colicky pains are better from bending over or passing a stool.

GYNECOLOGICAL PROBLEMS
- There may be long-standing problems with periods that are too early, too frequent, or too heavy.
- Periods are very distressing because of too-heavy bleeding.
- The flow is heavy, dark, and clotted.

- Cramping pains increase proportionally with the amount of menstrual flow.
- Bearing down, prolapse-type pains move across the lower abdomen and down into the upper thighs.
- Breasts are very sensitive during the period.
- All symptoms are worse during menstrual periods.
- During menopause there are exaggerated or heightened symptoms, such as migraines, headaches, flooding, hot flashes, and emotional problems such as depression.

JOINTS AND MUSCLES
- Persistent pain and stiffness in the back are caused by straining or exposure to cold, damp conditions. It is worse with initial movement after being still and improved by lying flat.
- Pains run from the back into the thighs, especially on the left side.
- There is muscular soreness with shooting pains, especially in the shoulders, base of the neck, and heels. These pains are eased by continued movement and made worse with damp and cold.
- Rheumatism is aggravated at night and during a period.

Symptoms are better

- after eating;
- with movement;
- in the fresh air;
- with warmth;
- with pressure.

Symptoms are worse

- during a period;

- with initial movement after rest;
- at night;
- with cold;
- with damp.

GELSEMIUM

Key Features

Gelsemium is indicated in the following circumstances.

- Symptoms develop slowly and insidiously, rather than violently and abruptly.
- There is a profound state of weariness and exhaustion.
- Limbs feel heavy and tremble on making an effort.
- Symptoms are flulike, with generalized aching, shivering, weariness, and chills running up and down the spine.

Emotions

Gelsemium may be required where the patient:

- is mentally and emotionally weary and wants to be left alone in peace;
- is listless and apathetic if anyone tries to cheer her up;
- is exhausted but also fearful and anxious, and in particular is afraid of the dark and anxious about death when depressed;
- is fearful in anticipation of any event that involves strain or effort;
- has difficulty in talking about emotions when depressed;
- is withdrawn, untalkative, and confused when anxious or stressed;

- has developed symptoms after a shock, fright, or distress following bad news or through anxiety linked to a coming stressful event.

Specific Symptoms

Gelsemium is indicated when the following symptoms occur.

HOT FLASHES
- Although the patient is shivery and chilly at times, hot flashes affect the head and face.
- She is very uncomfortable in a stuffy, overheated room.
- She feels anxious and unable to breathe when overheated.

SLEEP
- Although the patient is very drowsy during the day, sleep is very unrefreshing and disturbed.
- She wakes with a start, feeling anxious.
- If night sweats occur, they are drenching and exhausting.

HEADACHE
- Headaches are severe, with a bandlike sensation around the forehead.
- The headache may begin at the nape of the neck, spreading to the area above the eyes.
- Before the headache begins, there is often a distressing feeling of dizziness or unsteadiness in walking, with a sensation of being about to fall.
- Menopausal headaches are accompanied by giddiness, drowsiness, and difficulty in focusing the eyes.
- Pains are relieved by lying down and resting and made worse by warmth and standing. Some headaches are relieved by passing large quantities of urine.

APPETITE AND DIGESTION
- Diarrhea is painless but frequent, brought on by anxiety or nervous tension.

BLADDER AND KIDNEY PROBLEMS
- Stress incontinence occurs as a result of weakness or poor control over the sphincter muscle of the bladder.

JOINTS AND MUSCLES
- There are heavy, aching, dragging sensations in the arms and legs.

Symptoms are better

- with gentle, continued motion;
- headaches benefit from passing large amounts of urine;
- after perspiring.

Symptoms are worse

- in overheated, stuffy rooms;
- in bright sunlight;
- in damp, cold weather;
- when thinking about symptoms;
- midmorning.

HEPAR SULPHURIS CALCAREUM (HEPAR SULPH.)

Key Features

Hepar sulph. is indicated in the following circumstances.

- There is extreme sensitivity on mental, emotional, and physical levels.
- Wounds heal slowly or become infected very quickly.
- Discharges are offensive and yellow or greenish.
- Pains are characteristically splintering and sharp or bruised.
- The patient is extremely chilly, with a marked intolerance of cold air.

Emotions

Hepar sulph. may be required where the patient:

- is very irritable and bad-tempered when feeling ill;
- is dissatisfied and extremely difficult to please;
- is very sensitive to pain and discomfort and becomes quarrelsome as a result;
- becomes abusive as a result of hypersensitivity.

Specific Symptoms

Hepar sulph. is indicated when the following symptoms occur.

HEADACHE
- The head and scalp are very sensitive to cold.
- Sinus problems cause pains in cheekbones or at the root of the nose.
- Bursting pains are made worse by moving the head and relieved by warmth or tight pressure.

JOINTS AND MUSCLES
- Joints are painful, stiff, and swollen and are worse in cold weather.
- Joints are weak and easily dislocated, and the knees tremble when walking.

- Cramping pains occur in thigh and calf muscles and are severe at night.

Symptoms are better

- with warmth;
- in humid weather;
- after eating.

Symptoms are worse

- in cold winds or cold drafts;
- with light touch;
- when lying on the painful side;
- in the morning and evening;
- in winter.

IGNATIA

Key Features

Ignatia is often needed in times of great emotional trauma, distress, or grief. It is indicated in the following circumstances.

- Physical reactions often involve muscular spasms, such as hiccups, involuntary gulping, or twitching muscles. Constant sighing or yawning are also common symptoms.
- Contradictory symptoms are common, such as an empty feeling in the stomach that is not improved by eating, a severe sore throat that is relieved by swallowing solid food, or a persistent tickle in the throat that is made worse by coughing.
- Trembling and shaking may occur anywhere in the body.

Emotions

Ignatia may be required where the patient:

- is very distressed and emotionally traumatized but bottles things up rather than expressing distress openly and immediately, so a trivial issue may trigger floods of tears and uncontrollable bouts of sobbing;
- has rapid and violent mood swings, alternating between laughter and tears, or between a determination to be alone and a desperate longing for company and distraction;
- is oversensitive on physical and emotional levels, with a tendency to resent criticism or contradiction;
- is extremely sensitive to pain, noise, or strong smells.

Specific Symptoms

Ignatia is indicated when the following symptoms occur.

SLEEP
- Insomnia sets in on hearing bad news or following bereavement.
- Sleep is very light and easily disturbed, with a tendency to wake at the slightest noise.
- Jarring or jerking sensations occur when falling asleep.

HEADACHE
- The head is hot and heavy, with a feeling of dizziness or unsteadiness.
- A migraine-type headache occurs with bright zigzags in front of the eyes and difficulty in focusing.
- Migraines are relieved by vomiting but are much worse with movement or in a smoky atmosphere.

- Emotional stress or the shock of bereavement may trigger headaches.
- Spasmodic pains occur in the head, with a feeling as though a nail is being pushed into the side or back of the head.

DIGESTION AND APPETITE
- There is a bitter taste in the mouth and excess saliva.
- The patient hiccups frequently, and undigested food rises into the throat. Both are made worse from smoking or eating.
- There is a sinking feeling in the stomach, with a need to take a deep breath to obtain relief.
- There is a feeling of hunger and emptiness in the stomach from nerves, and this is not improved by eating.
- Feeling ill is accompanied by a craving for unusual or indigestible foods, such as acidic ingredients or heavy meals.
- Emotional strain causes constipation, with a frequent, ineffectual urge to pass a stool.
- Unusually, a hard stool is easier to pass than a soft one.
- Urgent, painless diarrhea follows an emotional shock.
- Hemorrhoids are worse for sitting and better for walking about. Pains are prickling and sticking, like little needles.

GYNECOLOGICAL PROBLEMS
- Hormonal imbalances arise as a result of emotional shock or trauma.
- Periods are very painful, with a dark-colored, offensive-smelling flow.
- Pains are relieved by movement, firm pressure, and lying down.

MUSCLES AND JOINTS
- Cramping, tingling pains extend from the back to the legs.

- Sciatic pains occur intermittently and are worse in cold weather and at night.

Symptoms are better

- after eating;
- with firm pressure on painful parts;
- with warmth;
- during distracting activities.

Symptoms are worse

- after taking sugar, coffee, or alcohol;
- with exposure to cigarette smoke or other strong smells;
- during emotional upsets;
- from yawning.

IPECACUANHA (IPECAC)

Key Features

Ipecac is indicated in the following circumstances.

- Persistent, severe nausea accompanies all complaints.
- There is a tendency to bleed easily and frequently.
- When exhausted, breathing is difficult.
- The patient is very sensitive to movement, which makes everything feel much worse.

Emotions

Ipecac may be required where the patient:

- is impatient and quarrelsome and finds fault with anything and everyone;
- is discontented and difficult to please;
- is extremely sensitive to noise, especially loud music;
- is suffering from illness brought on by anger and bottled-up emotion.

Specific Symptoms

Ipecac is indicated when the following symptoms occur.

APPETITE AND DIGESTION
- Awful, persistent nausea is not improved by anything, including vomiting.
- There is a nauseating sensation and an excess of saliva in the mouth.
- There is a constant urging to pass diarrhea-type stools, which are passed frequently and in large quantities.
- Diarrhea is severe and painful after eating an excessive amount of sugar or unripe fruit.

CYSTITIS AND KIDNEY PROBLEMS
- Shooting pains occur in the sides with constant desire to urinate.
- Urine is blood-streaked or contains a reddish sediment.
- Nausea and vomiting occur with cystitis or kidney disorders.

GYNECOLOGICAL PROBLEMS
- Spotting or intermittent bleeding occurs between periods.
- Menstrual flow is gushing, heavy, and bright red. Movement increases the amount of the flow.
- Bleeding is increased by chill or shock.
- Nausea, vomiting, and faintness accompany period pains.

- When periods are very heavy and exhausting, there may be a strong craving for fresh, open air.

Symptoms are better

- with firm pressure;
- in the fresh, open air;
- when resting with the eyes closed.

Symptoms are worse

- in extreme heat or cold;
- after eating;
- with a diet that involves regular meat intake;
- in dry or humid conditions;
- with movement;
- with light touch.

KALIUM CARBONICUM (KALI. CARB.)

Key Features

Kali. carb. is indicated in the following circumstances.

- Problems affect the right side of the body.
- The patient is very sensitive to cold.
- Pains are characteristically cutting, stitching, or stabbing wherever they occur in the body.
- Although the affected parts feel cold, the specific pain may be burning in character.
- Discomfort flits from place to place: once one area is soothed by warmth, pains pop up in another place.
- Anemia or fluid retention is present.

Emotions

Kali. carb. may be required where the patient:

- is physically exhausted, and therefore extremely irritable and on edge;
- has severe mood swings and is unable to cope with stress;
- is at odds with everyone and everything; craves company but cannot abide sympathy;
- is apathetic and lacks interest in anything;
- is hypersensitive to everything, especially loud noise;
- shakes and trembles after an emotional trauma or upset;
- is afraid of what will happen in the future, death, or ghosts.

Specific Symptoms

Kali. carb. is indicated when the following symptoms occur.

HEADACHE
- Frequent headaches occur as a result of persistent sinus problems.
- Burning pains are felt above the eyes or in the cheekbones.
- Head pains are much more intense from contact with cold and eased considerably by warmth and pressure.
- There is an instinctive desire to wrap up the head warmly as a way of avoiding inhaling cold air.

APPETITE AND DIGESTION
- Weak or sinking sensations in the stomach are increased rather than improved by eating.
- Discomfort and heavy feelings in the stomach are experienced after a meal.
- Heartburn and burning in the stomach are worse after cold drinks.

- Bloating comes on soon after eating, with severe belching and flatulence.
- Colicky, cramping pains are eased by bending over double and from contact with warmth.
- Constipation alternates with diarrhea.
- Large hemorrhoids that bleed easily give rise to burning pains that are eased by cool bathing (unlike burning pains elsewhere in the body).

CYSTITIS AND KIDNEY PROBLEMS
- Urine must be passed frequently.
- Burning pains occur during and after urination.
- Although there may be an urgent need to urinate, it may take a while before the flow starts.
- There is a general state of fluid retention and puffiness as a result of poor or sluggish kidney function.

GYNECOLOGICAL PROBLEMS
- There are troublesome cramping pains and chilliness before a period begins.
- There is persistent constipation during the menstrual period.
- Low back pain occurs with periods or prolapse.
- Weakness and diminished energy levels follow sexual intercourse.
- Flooding periods may persist, even after surgical techniques, such as dilatation and curettage (D and C), have been used.

JOINTS AND MUSCLES
- There is severe muscular weakness, with a tendency for the legs to "give way" without warning.
- Weakness and pain in the back are worse when walking and better when lying down.
- Back pain extends from the base of the spine to the thighs.

The discomfort may be worse before a period.
- Firm pressure to the painful area is very comforting and rest also helps.

Symptoms are better

- with warmth;
- during the day;
- when leaning forward.

Symptoms are worse

- from exposure to chill or cold;
- from contact with cold air or water;
- during changes in weather;
- on becoming overheated;
- after drinking coffee;
- in the early morning.

LACHESIS

Key Features

Lachesis is indicated in the following circumstances.

- Symptoms usually affect the left side of the body or start on the left and move gradually to the right.
- There is a strong dislike of clothing that is tight or constricting, especially around the neck.
- The skin may have a purple, mottled appearance, with a strong tendency to develop varicose veins or bruise easily.
- All symptoms are much worse on waking, and as a result there is a strong fear of falling asleep.

- Contact with heat makes everything worse, while cold drinks and exposure to fresh, cool air improve the situation.
- Because all symptoms are worse when periods are absent, menopause is an especially difficult time. As a result, there may be especially severe problems with hot flashes, depression, and general circulatory conditions such as thrombosis, phlebitis, and high blood pressure.

Emotions

Lachesis may be required where the patient:

- is full of energy and ideas but tends to suffer extreme mood swings;
- is emotionally unstable and sensitive, with symptoms worse before a period but improving as soon as the flow begins;
- is very much a "night person," with a tendency to experience a rush of creative ideas in the early hours and feel sluggish and fuzzy-headed the next morning as a result;
- has bouts of anxiety and depression alternating with anger, jealousy, and suspicion;
- is particularly anxious and depressed on waking;
- has surges of self-confidence and self-esteem alternating with extreme feelings of inadequacy and depression and periods of talkativeness alternating with silence and withdrawal;
- suffers from exhaustion and tiredness that are not improved by sleeping.

Specific Symptoms

Lachesis is indicated when the following symptoms occur.

HOT FLASHES
- Circulation is extremely unstable, with waves of heat traveling through the body.
- During a hot flash, the head may be very hot while the hands and feet remain cold.
- The patient is very sensitive to overheating, cannot tolerate warm, stuffy rooms, and craves cool, fresh air.
- Hot flashes are much worse when wearing tight clothing, especially about the neck.

SLEEP
- Sleep is disturbed by severe night sweats and anxiety.
- There is a dread of going to bed because of unpleasant sensations of disorientation on waking.
- The patient fears going to sleep because of a conviction that she may die in her sleep. This may be partly caused by feelings of suffocation or breathing problems that occur just as she is about to fall asleep. She may also experience a sensation of falling as she is losing consciousness which makes her wake with a start.
- The night may also be a difficult time because of a long-term fear of the supernatural, such as a fear of ghosts or the dead. These anxieties may surface with a vengeance at night.

HEADACHE
- Headaches are severe and left-sided and are worse when periods are absent.
- Head pains are relieved as soon as a discharge begins. This may either be a discharge that specifically relates to the

head, such as the onset of a runny nose or nosebleed, or a more general event, such as the onset of a menstrual period.

- Migraine-type headaches may be accompanied by a distressing dizziness, which is worse when the eyes are closed and better when lying down.

APPETITE AND DIGESTION

- Bloating and discomfort occur after eating. Both are made worse by clothes with a tight waistband that puts pressure around the waist.
- Troublesome constipation may set in, with hemorrhoids that are purple and bleed very easily.
- With constipation there is a feeling of a lump or plug in the rectum.
- There may be a history of severe pain from gallbladder problems.
- The patient prefers cool to warm drinks and may have a strong dislike of bread. Although there may be a craving for wine or milk, both of these may have a bad effect on the system.

GYNECOLOGICAL PROBLEMS

- There are long-term problems with the ovaries, especially on the left side. There may be a history of ovarian cysts.
- Severe pains occur before a period begins and are relieved as soon as the flow starts.
- Menstrual flow is very heavy and dark, often with large clots.
- Severe symptoms that resemble premenstrual syndrome occur once menopause is well under way, especially mood swings and emotional reactions.

Symptoms are better

- in the cool, fresh air;
- with cool drinks;
- at the onset of a period;
- with the appearance of a discharge;
- after moderate exercise.

Symptoms are worse

- with touch or constriction;
- on becoming overheated;
- when periods are delayed or absent;
- after sleep;
- on the left side;
- in spring;
- from drinking alcohol;
- after a warm bath.

LEDUM

Key Features

Ledum is indicated in the following circumstances.

- Although the patient is generally chilly, pains are relieved by contact with cool compresses or bathing in cold water.
- There are swollen, tight areas with fluid retention.
- Pains are sharp or stabbing. They shift about readily from one part to another or move from the lower limbs to the upper parts of the body.
- Wounds become quickly septic, and abscesses form readily.

Emotions

Ledum may be required where the patient:

- is dissatisfied and irritable with everything and everyone;
- is weepy when depressed and sighs between bouts of sobbing.

Headaches

- The patient dislikes covering the head when suffering from a headache.
- Pressing pains in the head are relieved from contact with cool air.

Specific Symptoms

Ledum is indicated when the following symptoms occur.

APPETITE AND DIGESTION
- There is nausea, with excess saliva in the mouth.
- Queasiness is worse when perspiring or when walking in the open air.
- Hemorrhoids occur, with anal fissure.

CYSTITIS AND KIDNEY PROBLEMS
- There is a constant need to urinate, and flow is interrupted.
- The urine has red deposits.
- Burning sensations are felt after urination.
- Joint problems are associated with passing large amounts of clear, colorless urine.

GYNECOLOGICAL PROBLEMS
- Menstrual flow is flooding and bright red.

- Although chilly during periods, the patient feels better for contact with cool air.

JOINTS AND MUSCLES
- Joint pains move from below upward.
- Joints are swollen, stiff, and hot but a normal color.
- All pains are relieved from contact with cool air or bathing. They are worse for warmth in general and for the specific heat of becoming warmed in bed at night.
- The small joints are especially affected, such as the fingers and toes. They are often knobbly and distorted from joint problems.
- Low back pain is worse from sitting still for too long.
- Stiff joints have to be bathed in cold water before they can be moved.

Symptoms are better

- with cold bathing;
- on contact with cool air;
- on applying cold compresses;
- with rest.

Symptoms are worse

- with warmth;
- on becoming warm in bed;
- at night;
- when wearing clothes that are too heavy or too warm;
- after drinking alcohol;
- when walking.

LYCOPODIUM

Key Features

Lycopodium is indicated in the following circumstances.

- Symptoms generally affect the right side of the body or move from right to left.
- Digestive problems are prominent, with a marked tendency to bloating, gurgling, and noisy flatulence.
- Lack of stamina results in rapid and frequent exhaustion after little physical effort.
- Although the patient is very chilly, stuffy or warm surroundings cause great distress and anxiety.
- All symptoms are much worse in the afternoons and improve in the evening. Energy levels are especially low and flagging at this time.

Emotions

Lycopodium may be required where the patient:

- presents an outward picture of confidence and competence, while inwardly racked with anxiety and fear of being unable to cope;
- adopts a veneer of sarcasm and haughtiness to disguise a strong sense of inadequacy, misleadingly appearing domineering and overconfident;
- is intellectually sharp with a tendency to appear detached and unemotional;
- is fearful and anxious when alone but dislikes company that is not of her own choosing or that becomes too demanding of her time and attention;

- is afraid of being seen to be a failure or inadequate to any given task, especially of speaking in public, which causes great anxiety before the event but usually turns out well;
- has an underlying fear of losing control, leading to anxieties over finances, death, or crowds, which are kept at bay by emotional and financial self-sufficiency but can appear out of proportion if this sense of security is threatened by ill-health;
- becomes rapidly confused and forgetful when stressed.

Specific Symptoms

Lycopodium is indicated when the following symptoms occur.

HOT FLASHES
- Hot flashes may be triggered by anxiety or emotional strain.
- Clammy perspiration may be left after a hot flash.
- Hot flashes are much worse for warm, airless surroundings or clothes that are too heavy or too warm.
- The patient feels hot and bothered if clothes are too tight, surroundings are too confined, or if someone approaches her.

SLEEP
- Disturbing dreams or nightmares occur, which involve sensations of restriction or suffocation.
- The patient has a disturbing feeling of falling on dropping to sleep, with jerking of the limbs.
- She is bad-tempered on waking, but her mood improves as she gets up and about.

HEADACHE
- Pains are felt in the temples as though the head is caught in a vice. The sensation is made worse by stuffy rooms and

lying down. They are improved by gentle movement and fresh, cool, open air.
- Low blood-sugar levels cause early-morning headaches that are quickly relieved by eating.
- Dizziness is worse on waking, talking, and eating or drinking.

APPETITE AND DIGESTION
- There is severe, recurrent heartburn and indigestion, with a sensation of acid rising up into the throat.
- Food may be eaten too quickly, with resulting gas and distension.
- Burning sensations in the stomach are soothed by warm drinks and made worse by cold.
- The patient sits down to a meal feeling hungry, becomes rapidly full after eating a few mouthfuls, and leaves the table but feels hungry again after an hour or so.
- The abdomen tends to rumble, gurgle, and swell, and there is a need to pass wind frequently. This problem is often associated with liver and gallbladder disorders.
- Constipation alternates with diarrhea when stress levels are high.
- Digestive problems are made worse by eating beans, peas, and cabbage.

CYSTITIS AND KIDNEY PROBLEMS
- Pains in the sides are relieved after urination.
- There is a frequent need to pass large amounts of pale urine.
- If bladder or kidney infection is present, urine is likely to be very concentrated. Upon examination, it may also contain a sediment that looks like red sand or brick dust.
- There is frequently a strong desire to urinate at short intervals during the night.

- If there is infection in the kidneys, it is likely to be right-sided.

GYNECOLOGICAL PROBLEMS
- Severe depression and irritability occur with premenstrual syndrome.
- An odd sensation is felt, as though gas is moving through the vagina.
- Periods may be irregular and heavy. The flow is likely to be dark and to contain large clots.

MUSCLES AND JOINTS
- Severe, tearing pains move from the right side of the neck to the shoulder, arm, and fingers.
- "Restless legs" at night disturb or interfere with sleep.
- Persistent back pain is soothed by warmth and made worse by movement.
- Knees are weak and feel as though they are about to give way.
- Swelling and soreness in joints are relieved by gentle movement.

Symptoms are better

- from gentle exercise in the fresh, open air;
- with warm food or drinks;
- after loosening a tight waistband;
- with moderate warmth;
- with distraction.

Symptoms are worse

- in cold weather;
- with cold food or drinks;

- on becoming overheated;
- with pressure or the weight of heavy clothing;
- with too much physical effort;
- on waking from sleep;
- at around 4:00 to 8:00 P.M.
- when unoccupied.

MERCURIUS SOLUBIS (MERC. SOL.)

Key Features

Merc. sol. is indicated in the following circumstances.

- There is a terrible physical and mental restlessness that is very much worse at night.
- All discharges, such as saliva, perspiration, and mucus, are increased.
- Extreme exhaustion sets in, often as a result of a severe anemic state.
- Fluid retention of the face, fingers, feet, and ankles is common.
- There is a marked tendency to persistent or severe swelling of the glands in the neck, armpits, or groin.
- Although the patient is basically chilly, any variation in temperature causes great uneasiness, discomfort, and restlessness.

Emotions

Merc. sol. may be required where the patient:

- is very agitated and restless and cannot stay still for any length of time;

- suffers mental and emotional symptoms that are much worse at night;
- has panic attacks for no apparent reason, with a desire to run away or escape;
- is confused and has a weak memory, especially for the names of people or places;
- becomes very apathetic and indifferent;
- feels rushed and compelled to do things in a great hurry.

Specific Symptoms

Merc. sol. is indicated when the following symptoms occur.

HOT FLASHES
- Panic attacks occur, with hot flashes of heat that affect the face and head, even though the rest of the body remains very chilly.
- Hot flashes cause profuse perspiration, leaving behind a sensation of shivering and clammy coldness.
- Hot flashes may alternate with bouts of extreme chilliness.

SLEEP
- All symptoms are very much worse at night, especially anxiety.
- There is severe insomnia or a disturbed sleep pattern.
- The patient wakes from sleep with a start, covered in a profuse sweat.
- Palpitations and anxiety at night may follow nightmares or disturbing dreams.

APPETITE AND DIGESTION
- Feelings of nausea occur, with excess saliva in the mouth.
- The tongue has a characteristic sensation of being swollen or enlarged.

- Recurrent, large, painful ulcers may be present in the mouth.
- There is an offensive taste in the mouth or odor to the breath.
- Acidity and gastric upsets are made worse from bending forward.
- Stomach upsets give rise to a persistent metallic taste.
- The patient dislikes meat, fat, and butter. Stomach upsets may follow eating foods that contain a great deal of sugar.

CYSTITIS AND KIDNEY PROBLEMS
- The patient has a constant, urgent need to pass small quantities of urine, day and night.
- There is severe burning during and after urination.
- The urine is acrid and burning.

GYNECOLOGICAL PROBLEMS
- Stinging or burning pains accompany ovarian problems.
- There is a greenish, irritating vaginal discharge that is worse at night or when urinating.
- Itching around the entrance to the vagina is soothed by cool bathing.

JOINTS AND MUSCLES
- Muscles are stiff and painful in the neck and back, with burning, low back pain that extends to the thighs.
- There is a feeling of restlessness and aching in the bones that is especially severe at night.
- "Restless legs" make it impossible to find a comfortable, restful spot, especially when warm in bed at night.
- Joints are stiff, painful, swollen, and pale, and feel worse for exposure to heat or chill.
- Cramping and stiffness in the hands make fine movements difficult.

Symptoms are better

- when resting in a moderate, constant temperature.

Symptoms are worse

- with extreme changes of temperature;
- at night;
- on becoming warm in bed;
- with exposure to chill or cold drafts;
- during the evening;
- when lying on the right side;
- after eating;
- with perspiring;
- when touched.

NATRUM MURIATICUM (NATRUM MUR.)

Key Features

Natrum mur. is indicated in the following circumstances.

- It is strongly indicated for symptoms of hormone imbalance, including fluid retention, mood swings, migraines or headaches that occur before, during, or after periods, or menopausal headaches.
- Dryness is a central feature, especially relating to the tone and texture of the skin and lips. A crack in the center of the bottom lip and a tendency to develop cold sores after exposure to sunlight are important features.

- Allergies frequently occur, with a particular tendency to hay fever, allergic rhinitis, prickly heat, urticaria (hives), or stress-related rashes.
- Hot sunlight or warm, stuffy surroundings are not tolerated at all well. Symptoms that may be aggravated or brought on by becoming overheated include headaches, skin eruptions, and hot flashes.
- There is a tendency for the patient to be withdrawn, depressed and reserved, with a marked dislike of attention and sympathy.
- The patient is easily exhausted and tired, especially in the mornings.

Emotions

Natrum mur. may be required where the patient:

- becomes ill after grief, bereavement, or bitter disappointment in a close relationship, where emotions have been bottled up or repressed;
- finds it difficult to express emotion, especially by crying, which only happens in private if at all, since crying in public is seen as embarrassing or a sign of weakness;
- though unhappy, dislikes expressions of sympathy or physical affection, since they may promote an undesired bout of weeping;
- is reserved and self-contained, with a definite dislike of revealing emotion or losing control of her feelings;
- is afraid of being robbed or is anxious in narrow or closed spaces;
- has moods that alternate between sadness and euphoria or overexcitability;
- though reserved and withdrawn, becomes resentful and lonely if feeling ignored or overlooked;

- is easily startled and frightened by unexpected or loud noises.

Specific Symptoms
Natrum mur. is indicated when the following symptoms occur.

HOT FLASHES
- Pulsating sensations and hot flashes rise without warning to the chest and head, while the legs stay cool.
- Palpitations may accompany a sense of being hot and bothered.

SLEEP
- It is difficult to get to sleep, or the patient wakes frequently from brooding on unpleasant thoughts.
- Night sweats occur during the later part of the night.

HEADACHE
- Headaches may come on as a result of low blood-sugar levels if a meal is delayed.
- Pains may be one-sided or affect the front of the head, causing nausea, vomiting, and a pale, pinched look.
- The head feels as though it is about to burst from throbbing pains. These are relieved by keeping the eyes as still as possible, lying down, vomiting, and sleeping.
- Migraines are preceded by tingling and numbness of the lips, tongue, and nose. A zigzag aura may also appear in front of the eyes before the headache starts.

APPETITE AND DIGESTION
- The mouth and lips are dry and tend to get recurrent cold sores or ulcers.
- Although the abdomen is full of gas, it is more comfortable when the waistband of clothes is tightened.

- There is a heavy feeling in the stomach, and the digestion is slow or sluggish.
- There may be either a craving for or dislike of salt and bread. Thirst may be very marked for large quantities of water.
- If the stomach is upset, the tongue takes on a characteristically "mapped" appearance, with shiny areas that look as though the surface of the tongue has been removed.
- Constipation may result from dry stools that are difficult to pass, with the added complication of hemorrhoids or an anal fissure or crack.

GYNECOLOGICAL PROBLEMS
- All symptoms may be worse during or toward the end of a menstrual period.
- Periods may be too early and heavy or delayed and scanty.
- Heavy, muscular contractions or back pain may accompany the menstrual flow, with or without a prolapse being present.
- If there is a prolapse, the discomfort will be worse on getting up in the morning, and relieved by sitting down with the legs crossed. The low back pain associated with a prolapse is eased by applying a firm support to the hollow of the back when seated.
- Dryness and painful sensitivity of the vagina may lead to a complete aversion to intercourse.
- Vaginal yeast infections and cystitis may also occur periodically, as a result of poor lubrication of the membranes around the genital area.

JOINTS AND MUSCLES
- Backache may emerge as a reaction to emotional stress.

Symptoms are better

- when alone;

- from contact with cool air, or cool bathing;
- from skipping meals;
- with gentle exercise;
- when resting;
- with tight clothes;
- in sea air (but this can also aggravate symptoms).

Symptoms are worse

- when overheated or exposed to strong sunlight;
- during or at the end of a period;
- with extreme changes of temperature;
- with overexertion;
- with mental, emotional, or physical stress;
- midmorning;
- with attention and sympathy;
- in sea air (but this can also improve symptoms).

NUX VOMICA

Key Features

Nux vomica is indicated in the following circumstances.

- There are signs of workaholism, with resulting high anxiety or stress levels, disturbed sleep pattern, digestive problems, and recurrent headaches.
- Additional problems may arise as a result of a high-pressured lifestyle, including a tendency to rely on alcohol, stimulants, sedatives, painkillers, and cigarettes as a way of coping.
- Oversensitivity on physical and emotional levels leads to irritability with an extreme intolerance of pain.

185

- Those who respond well to Nux vomica are very chilly by nature with severe dislike of cold or drafty conditions.
- Pains are spasmodic, cramping, and constricting.

Emotions

Nux vomica may be required where the patient:

- is tense, nervous, and overstressed under pressure;
- is very irritable and inclined to pick a quarrel when out of sorts;
- is fastidious and overattentive to detail, setting high standards that become a strain to live up to;
- tolerates contradiction and consolation very badly, often reacting impatiently and aggressively;
- overdoes everything, demanding 101 percent from everyone, including herself, which leads to "burnout"—mental, emotional, and physical exhaustion;
- has fits of anger that may result in violence, with shouting, screaming, and objects being hurled to the ground;
- feels generally better after an outburst or shouting match;
- is irritable and oversensitive to cold, light, noise, pain, touch, and food as a result of an overloaded system.

Specific Symptoms

Nux vomica is indicated when the following symptoms occur.

SLEEP
- Too many ideas buzz around in the head, preventing sleep.
- Sleep is light and catnapping and is easily disturbed by the slightest sound.
- The patient wakes in the early hours feeling alert and ready to get up, falls back to sleep after a while, and wakes

feeling "hungover" and headachy when it is time to get out of bed.

- Sleep problems may occur because of an addiction to caffeine.

HEADACHE

- The classic "morning-after" sensation, with dizziness, heavy feeling at the back of the head, nausea, and sensitivity to strong smells such as tobacco or coffee is worse on waking, and from movement of any kind. Warmth, resting in bed, and quiet surroundings are all soothing.
- The head is extremely sensitive to cold, drafty conditions.

APPETITE AND DIGESTION

- With stomach upsets, there is a nasty taste in the mouth and the tongue is coated and discolored.
- Digestive problems occur after drinking too much alcohol or eating a mixture of rich food.
- A hot flash may occur immediately after eating a meal, which may be quickly followed by feeling sleepy and drowsy.
- The patient becomes quickly bloated around the waist or feels faint or uncomfortably hot after eating rich food with plenty of alcohol in stuffy surroundings.
- Nervous indigestion occurs when she is stressed, with a heavy sensation in the stomach and a queasy feeling after eating.
- Heartburn may be relieved by vomiting.
- Cramping pains are eased by lying or sitting down.
- Gallbladder disorders lead to severe pains that feel worse for movement or pressure and better for warmth.
- There is habitual constipation, with a great deal of fruitless urging.

- "Bashful stool" syndrome occurs: as soon as a stool begins to be expelled, it slips back into the rectum.
- A temporary sense of relief is felt once a bowel movement has been achieved.
- Long-term reliance on laxatives leads to a cycle of constipation followed by diarrhea, which ends in further problems with constipation. Sluggish or infrequent bowel movements may also result from overfrequent use of painkillers, especially those that contain codeine.
- Very painful, itchy hemorrhoids are worse during times of stress, and after a bowel movement. They also tend to bleed very readily.

CYSTITIS AND KIDNEY PROBLEMS
- Right-sided kidney pains are felt, with difficulty in urinating.
- Burning sensations occur with bladder infections such as cystitis and are especially severe at night.
- Itching or burning is felt when urinating.

JOINTS AND MUSCLES
- Rheumatic, muscular pains and spasms feel aching, bruised, or sharp and extend from the nape of the neck to the base of the spine.
- Joints and muscles are stiff and immobile, especially on initial movement after waking.
- A weak feeling in the joints is aggravated by cold conditions and exertion.
- Cramping pains occur in bed at night, especially affecting the calf muscles.

Symptoms are better

- after unbroken sleep;

- in peaceful surroundings;
- as the day goes on;
- in humid conditions.

Symptoms are worse

- on waking;
- after disturbed sleep;
- after eating;
- from overuse of alcohol, tobacco, painkillers or sleeping tablets;
- with touch;
- when stressed;
- in cold, drafty conditions.

PHOSPHORUS

Key Features

Phosphorus is indicated in the following circumstances.

- Those who benefit most are usually subject to periods of rapidly developing exhaustion and weakness, often as a result of an underlying anemic state.
- A general lack of stamina leads to bursts of energy, enthusiasm, and sociability, rapidly followed by apathy, indifference, and introversion.
- A fundamental state of anxiety leads to the emergence of a host of fears when ill. This "free-floating" form of anxiety attaches itself to any current issue that may have the potential to cause problems.
- Sensations are characteristically burning wherever they are felt in the body. This is linked to circulatory instability,

causing alternating hot flashes of heat and chilliness.
- A general tendency to suffer from fluid retention may give rise to puffiness of the hands, ankles, feet, and eyelids.

Emotions

Phosphorus may be required where the patient:

- is enthusiastic, extroverted, and lively when feeling well but rapidly becomes bad-tempered or withdrawn when burned out;
- is quickly moved to tears when physically, mentally, or emotionally exhausted;
- is very sensitive to the feelings of others and inclined to empathize to a degree that may drain her own emotional reserves;
- is extremely open to new ideas and interests and may have a particular fascination with the paranormal due to her sensitivity to others;
- responds well to displays of physical affection and always feels much better for physical contact, such as having a massage;
- is sensitive and responsive to sensory stimuli such as perfume, color, light, music, and touch;
- needs attention, sympathy, and displays of affection from others when unwell and feels low and anxious if alone or neglected;
- is afraid of the dark, thunderstorms, being alone, spiders, and in particular, illness, but these fears can be diminished by reassurance from someone she trusts.

Specific Symptoms

Phosphorus is indicated when the following symptoms occur.

HOT FLASHES
- Hot flashes may be preceded by anxiety and panic.
- Although the patient is generally chilly, when a hot flash occurs there is a sudden sensation of internal or external burning.
- Sudden alterations in blood flow may produce the effect of an overheated head and torso, while the legs and feet feel icy cold.

SLEEP
- Sleep is restless, and there is a sense of feeling tired and unrefreshed on waking.
- Palpitations and anxious uneasiness are worse for sleeping on the left side.
- Heavy night sweats occur during the second half of the night.

HEADACHE
- Circulatory irregularities result in dizziness and unsteadiness on getting up quickly from a sitting or lying position. These symptoms may also be brought on by eating, turning the head quickly, or stooping and may frequently occur if there is low blood pressure.
- Headaches occur with burning pains that are relieved by cool applications and sitting up and are made worse by warm surroundings and lying down.
- Headaches that occur as a result of low blood-sugar levels are quickly relieved by eating a small amount of food.
- A hot flash often accompanies a headache, spreading from the head and face over the whole body.

APPETITE AND DIGESTION
- Burning pains in the stomach occur with a queasy, weak sensation. This feeling often comes on soon after eating and is relieved by cold food or drink but aggravated by warm food or drink.

- Cool foods and drinks are initially very soothing, but the burning sensation returns as the stomach contents become warmed during the process of digestion.
- There is constant nausea, with a feeling of fullness and burning pains in the stomach.
- Belching causes more discomfort than relief and brings an unpleasant taste of food into the mouth.
- Cravings for salty and highly spiced food such as curries, chillies, or Thai dishes are common. Dislikes include milky puddings, boiled milk, beer, fish, tea, and coffee.
- Rumbling and gurgling extend from the stomach down the length of the gut.
- Hemorrhoids bleed easily, with a passage of bright red blood with each stool.

CYSTITIS AND KIDNEY PROBLEMS
- There is a constant desire to pass very concentrated amounts of urine, with burning sensations.
- Urine may be discolored with a fatty-looking deposit on the surface. It may also include traces of blood.
- A tendency to diabetes may be detected if there is a marked increase in thirst, with a large amount of pale urine being passed more frequently than usual.

GYNECOLOGICAL PROBLEMS
- Sadness, tearfulness, and severe shifts in mood occur before a period is due.
- When a period arrives, it may be intensely heavy, with bright red, clotted flow.
- There may be a general sensitivity of the area around the vagina, with a heavy, burning discharge.

JOINTS AND MUSCLES
- There is stiffness and discomfort in the neck and back

muscles that is much worse in the morning.
- The fingers are stiff and numb, and there is a general sense of weakness in the arms and legs.
- There is discomfort in the hip joints, with a general soreness of the spine that is worse for the least touch.
- There are burning sensations in the spine at night, while the legs and knees feel very cold.

Symptoms are better

- with reassurance and attention;
- with warmth;
- from eating small amounts regularly;
- after uninterrupted sleep;
- with massage.

Symptoms are worse

- on becoming damp;
- with cold;
- when lying on the left side;
- in darkness;
- when alone;
- in crowded places;
- at heights;
- with overexcitement or stimulation;
- during thunderstorms.

PULSATILLA

Key Features

Pulsatilla is indicated in the following circumstances.

- There is changeability on both physical and emotional levels: moods change rapidly and pains shift constantly.
- Although the patient is basically chilly, there is a marked intolerance of heated, airless rooms, and a strong desire for cool, fresh air.
- Pulsatilla is often indicated at times of hormonal instability, provided the general symptoms agree: for example, at puberty, during menopause, or premenstrually.
- The circulatory system is sluggish or inefficient, leading to varicose veins, chilblains, or very cold hands and feet.
- All symptoms are much better for movement and worse for lying in bed or resting. Great benefit is derived from exercising gently in the open air, since this stimulates a sluggish circulation.
- Symptoms tend to affect the right side of the body.

Emotions

Pulsatilla may be required where the patient:

- has changeable moods with a tendency to burst into tears very easily;
- feels much better after a good cry in sympathetic company;
- craves attention and sympathy when feeling down and feels worse when alone and feeling neglected;
- is gregarious and eager for company;
- is easily persuaded to change her opinion or finds it difficult to make a decision, because of low self-confidence or poor self-esteem;
- is afraid of the dark, being alone, going insane, or crowds and open spaces.

Specific Symptoms

Pulsatilla is indicated when the following symptoms occur.

Checklist of Homeopathic Remedies

HOT FLASHES

- The patient constantly alternates between feeling too hot and too cold, so rarely feels comfortable.
- Although she is chilly much of the time, being in a stuffy or overheated room is unbearable, causing faintness, hot flashes, and dizziness.
- She always feels more comfortable if a window is open, giving ready access to fresh, open air.
- Palpitations occur with hot flashes, especially after a heavy meal.

SLEEP

- The patient cannot stand heavy bedcovers because of a tendency to become overheated at night. She pushes the covers off until she cools down, becomes too chilly, and then has to haul them back up again.
- Although she is sleepy when going to bed, sleep is disturbed and fitful. She wakes in the early hours of the morning feeling very restless and has great difficulty in getting back to sleep again.
- Night sweats occur frequently, with heavy perspiration and a sensation that waves of heat are coursing through the body. Sweats are especially pronounced on the face.

HEADACHE

- Headaches are brought on by eating a diet that is too rich or fatty or by surroundings that are stuffy, airless, or overheated.
- Headaches may frequently be connected to menstrual problems or digestive upsets.
- Dizziness accompanies headaches and is especially pronounced when getting up after sitting or lying down, and when walking outdoors.

APPETITE AND DIGESTION

- Although the mouth is dry, there is no thirst.
- Indigestion and heavy feelings in the stomach come on an hour or two after eating.
- Belching causes food to "repeat." Burning sensations are worse for eating warm food and better for cool drinks.
- Stomach pains and distension are worse each evening and after eating rich foods.
- The patient craves rich, fatty foods and pastries that upset the stomach. She dislikes milk, butter, and pork.
- Constipation is troublesome, with a sensation that the bowel has not been completely emptied.
- Diarrhea is brought on from chill, iced drinks, ice cream, or too much fruit.
- Hemorrhoids are itchy, painful, and protruding. They are worse for warmth and better for coolness.

CYSTITIS AND KIDNEY PROBLEMS

- Stress incontinence occurs, with leaking of urine that is worse from coughing, walking, or sitting.
- There is a frequent desire to urinate at night, especially when lying on the back.
- Passing urine is painful, with a sore sensation afterward.
- There is irritation and inflammation of the bladder, causing a strong and frequent urge to urinate, which becomes very distressing if there is any delay in emptying the bladder.
- There may be a history of urinary problems in pregnancy.

GYNECOLOGICAL PROBLEMS

- Vaginal discharge is bland, thick, creamy, or greenish. It may be accompanied by irritation or persistent itching of the vaginal area.
- Distressing breast tenderness with period.

- Periods may be delayed and very short in duration, with a scanty flow.
- During menopause there is a constant sensation that a period is imminent.
- Prolapse occurs with a severe back pain that is worse with heat and better with gentle movement.

JOINTS AND MUSCLES
- The arms and legs feel heavy, bruised, and sore.
- Pains are changeable and shift rapidly from place to place.
- There are heavy feelings in the legs that are worse by day and give way to aching sensations at night.
- Curvature of the spine gives rise to pains in the lower back.
- Pain, stiffness, and swelling in the joints are worse with warmth, resting, and initial movement after being still. They are relieved by cool applications, continued gentle exercise, and firm pressure.

Symptoms are better

- in the fresh, open air;
- in cool conditions;
- with gentle exercise;
- with firm pressure to the painful area;
- with cool food and drinks;
- after uncovering;
- with attention and sympathy;
- after having a good cry.

Symptoms are worse

- in humid conditions;
- with heat;
- from a lack of fresh air;

- with clothes or covers that are too heavy or too warm;
- when resting;
- in the evening or at night;
- when feeling neglected;
- when alone.

RHUS TOXICONDENDRON (RHUS TOX.)

Key Features

Rhus tox. is indicated in the following circumstances.

- Pains are much worse when resting and keeping still and better with continued movement, provided it doesn't become overtaxing.
- Symptoms are generally relieved by warm bathing and are worse in cold, damp conditions.
- Blistery eruptions tend to emerge on the skin such as cold sores, eczema, and urticaria (hives). Rhus tox. is also a major remedy for chicken pox, with its characteristic raised, blistery, maddeningly itchy rash.
- All symptoms become more severe at night. This includes the depression that accompanies distressing physical ailments.
- A severe physical and mental restlessness sets in when unwell, especially at night.

Emotions

Rhus tox. may be required where the patient:

- is anxious in bed at night and feels weepy and in despair;
- has mental and emotional symptoms that become more severe when resting;

- has a long-term fear about being poisoned and is therefore very suspicious of taking any medicines;
- is restless, irritable, and nervous, being specifically anxious about her job, family, or financial affairs or generally uneasy about what the future holds in store;
- broods on distressing or unpleasant memories from the past, especially at night when there are few distractions.

Specific Symptoms

Rhus tox. is indicated when the following symptoms occur.

SLEEP
- The patient is restless and uncomfortable at night. The second half of the night is especially distressing.
- Sleep is fitful, disturbed, and restless. When asleep, she often dreams of activities that involve great effort and exertion.
- Night sweats are severe and made much worse by taking a warm drink.
- She wakes from sleep trembling and perspiring heavily.

HEADACHE
- Severe headaches come on during or after exposure to a chill. They are worse for moving the head, and the pains affect the front of the head.
- Severe pains affect the base of the skull with a painful sensitivity of the scalp. This type of headache may be brought on by a fit of frustration or anger.
- Migraine-type headaches are improved considerably by taking a walk in the fresh air.

APPETITE AND DIGESTION
- The tongue is sensitive, coated, and discolored, with a characteristic red triangular tip.

- Eating patterns are irregular: a strong aversion to eating alternates with short bouts of ravenous hunger.
- Cramping, colicky pains are relieved by gentle movement or by bending over double.
- An unquenchable thirst for cold drinks is especially severe at night.
- The patient craves cold milk and sweet foods and dislikes meat and bread.

JOINTS AND MUSCLES
- Joints are stiff, swollen, and painful and are worse when keeping still and with initial movement after rest but better for continued, gentle exercise.
- Pains develop during damp, cold weather or after exposure to cold, drafty conditions.
- Restlessness accompanies joint pains, resulting in constant movement.
- Stiffness in the neck is worse on waking and with initial movement.
- Tingling in the shin bones is worse from contact with heat.
- Aches, pains, and muscular weakness occur as a result of exercising too vigorously or too long.

Symptoms are better

- after a hot bath;
- with warmth;
- in dry, warm weather;
- when wrapped up snugly;
- with gentle exercise that is not continued for too long.

Symptoms are worse

- in cold, wet weather;

- with cold winds;
- when resting;
- when standing still;
- with initial movement after a night's rest;
- with overexertion;
- during the evening;
- at night.

RUTA

Key Features

Ruta has a special affinity with aches and pains in the bones and joints. It is indicated in the following circumstances.

- It is of specific value when an injury has been sustained to the periosteum (the membranous sheath that covers the bones). If the periosteum has been damaged or bruised from a fall, pains can continue for an extended period, long after the superficial bruising has healed.
- There is a tremendous restlessness and difficulty in sitting still for any substantial time.
- There is a general chilliness, with a desire to keep as warm as possible.
- The patient is drowsy by day and wakeful at night.
- She yawns frequently and has a constant urge to stretch the limbs.

Emotions

Ruta may be required where the patient:

- is anxious and restless, especially at twilight;

- is weepy and depressed about recent events;
- is irritable and quarrelsome when joints are painful.

Specific Symptoms

Ruta is indicated when the following symptoms occur.

JOINTS AND MUSCLES
- Bruised pains in the spine are much worse when sitting down.
- Pain in the lower back is relieved by lying on the back.
- Weak joints give way when going up or down steps or when getting up from a sitting position.
- Bruised sensations in the thighs make walking difficult.
- Pains are especially common in the knuckles, wrists, knees, and ankles.
- There is a feeling of constant restlessness in the legs: she doesn't know where to put them to get comfortable.

Symptoms are better

- with gentle movement indoors;
- with warmth.

Symptoms are worse

- when resting;
- when lying on the painful area;
- when walking in the fresh air;
- when stooping;
- with touch.

Sepia

Key Features

Sepia is one of the major remedies for gynecological disorders. It is indicated in the following circumstances.

- Energy levels are low, and there is a general feeling of gloom and depression.
- There is a lack of interest in anything that demands motivation or enthusiasm.
- Symptoms are drooping or sagging in nature, especially with problems such a prolapse or backache.
- Although the patient is generally exhausted, there is a marked improvement in energy levels and well-being after vigorous exercise, if the initial effort can be made.
- Many of the symptoms that respond well to Sepia are caused by unstable or low blood-sugar levels. There may therefore be a history of problems with nausea and dizziness related to the menstrual cycle or during pregnancy when blood-sugar levels can be especially erratic.
- Sluggish or inefficient circulation results in a tendency to have varicose veins, hemorrhoids, and irregular distribution of heat in the body.
- A sensation of a ball or lump can occur anywhere in the body.

Emotions

Sepia may be required where the patient:

- is irritable and bad-tempered when overwhelmed with emotional or domestic demands and feels unable to cope when illness sets in, even though she normally deals well with day-to-day affairs;

- is indifferent or averse to her sexual partner, with a total lack of enthusiasm about sex, largely because of a profound state of physical, emotional, and mental exhaustion;
- is introverted, with a deep, black depression and lack of interest in everything;
- is anxious and agitated when unable to cope and ends up screaming at her family out of frustration, wanting to run away and escape from ties and demands;
- feels such despair that it is impossible to talk about her problems without bursting into tears;
- suffers emotional symptoms that are worse before a period or during menopause.

Specific Symptoms

Sepia is indicated when the following symptoms occur.

HOT FLASHES
- Hot flashes are followed by drenching sweats. When the flash is present, she feels as though she is immersed in hot water.
- Sweats may be brought on by very little physical effort.
- A hot flash may frequently occur with very little redness of the skin.
- Hot flashes move upward from the lower limbs to the neck and head.

SLEEP
- The patient is drowsy during the day and the evening but has great difficulty falling asleep at night.
- She remains awake for ages or wakes frequently during the night. As a result, she feels as though she has not slept at all when it is time to get up.
- She is uncomfortable and restless in bed, with distressing

night sweats that affect the head, chest, thighs, and back.

HEADACHE
- Headaches are one-sided and severe, with throbbing or shooting pains that move in an upward or outward direction.
- Migraine headaches are accompanied by nausea at the sight or smell of food, especially cooking smells.
- Headache is relieved by sleeping and by fresh, open air. It is made worse by movement, thunder, light, and noise.
- Unpleasant giddy sensations occur as a result of poor circulation or low blood pressure. They are especially severe in the morning or when walking.

APPETITE AND DIGESTION
- There is an unpleasant, weak, sinking sensation in the stomach, associated with faintness and dizziness.
- Nausea that is present on waking is relieved by eating or taking a hot drink.
- The patient craves condiments such as pickles and vinegar and spicy foods. She dislikes meat, milk, and meat fat.
- There is a gnawing hunger that is not eased by eating.
- Stools are difficult to pass, whether they are soft or hard and dry.
- There is a sensation of pressure or swelling in the rectum that is not eased by passing a stool.
- Hemorrhoids bleed easily and give rise to sharp, stitching pains that shoot upward.

CYSTITIS AND KIDNEY PROBLEMS
- A tense or pressured feeling in the bladder causes the sensation of frequently needing to urinate.
- Although there is an urgent and constant desire to urinate, very little may be passed each time. These sensations are especially troublesome and distressing at night.

- Urine may leak at night due to poor bladder tone.
- Urine is discolored and unpleasant-smelling and may contain a yellow or red sandy sediment. This type of sediment suggests a high content of uric acid, with an attendant risk of developing joint problems and kidney stones.

GYNECOLOGICAL PROBLEMS
- All symptoms tend to be much worse before periods, owing to a general tendency toward hormonal imbalance.
- Deep depression and irritability are especially severe before a period.
- Marked aversion to sexual activity is often the result of painful dryness of the vagina. This, in turn, leads to frequent vaginal and bladder infections, such as yeast infections and cystitis.
- Discharge may be irritating, yellow, green, and sometimes offensive smelling.
- Severe itching accompanies dryness and sensitivity of the vagina, which is much worse when walking.
- Erosion of the cervix may be present, with tremendous sensitivity and discomfort on examination.
- Uterine prolapse occurs with the sensation that everything is about to fall out of the pelvic cavity. When this feeling is very severe, the only position that gives relief is sitting with the legs firmly crossed. Standing and walking make it much worse.

JOINTS AND MUSCLES
- There may be severe, dragging back pain associated with a prolapse or menstrual problems. It is relieved by firm pressure to the painful area.
- There are heavy, weak sensations in the legs, which "give way" when walking, especially at the knees.

- Painful, puffy swelling of the knees is worse when going down stairs.
- Bruised pains in the joints are worse after resting.

Symptoms are better

- from vigorous exercise in the open air;
- when warm in bed;
- with eating regularly;
- after sleep;
- with firm pressure;
- when the legs are raised.

Symptoms are worse

- when sitting still (except for backache and prolapse);
- before a period;
- with emotional demands;
- before a thunderstorm;
- after going too long without food.

SILICA

Key Features

Silica is indicated in the following circumstances.

- Conditions develop slowly, insidiously, and progressively over a long period.
- Although subject to flashes of heat, those who benefit from Silica are usually chilly by nature.
- Illness may have been precipitated by a stressful, shocking, or upsetting event. The reaction to this distressing episode, however, may take a while to come to the surface.

- The patient is constantly tired and subject to regular infection with colds due to poor functioning of the immune system. As a result, sore throats and enlarged, painful glands are a common occurrence.
- Wounds and cuts tend to heal slowly, often leaving a scar behind. There is also a tendency for skin abrasions and eruptions to become infected rapidly, producing a thin, clear, pussy discharge.

Emotions

Silica may be required where the patient:

- is anxious, timid, and indecisive and finds it difficult to take a firm stance on anything;
- develops fixed ideas as a way of compensating for lack of decisiveness in other areas;
- lacks confidence and has difficulty in concentrating or fixing attention;
- is afraid of failure, loud noises, being unable to cope, and sharp objects such as needles;
- finds thinking and talking an enormous effort when she is "burnt out," and this leads to a profound depression;
- lacks drive, initiative, and dynamism when unwell, although at her best she is methodical, conscientious, and steadily productive.

Specific Symptoms

Silica is indicated when the following symptoms occur.

HOT FLASHES
- Although generally chilly, hot flashes may occur rapidly, especially if agitated or anxious.

- Perspires easily on the forehead, scalp, and neck. The feet also tend to be very sweaty.

SLEEP
- Sleep is disturbed and there may be a history of sleep-walking.
- Drenching night sweats are common.

HEADACHE
- Headaches are right-sided, with a distressing rush of blood to the head.
- Recurrent headaches begin at the back of the head and extend over the eyes. Pains are severe and bursting.
- Headaches are eased by keeping the head well wrapped up and by applying pressure and warm compresses to the forehead. They are intensified by chill, mental effort, light, noise, and moving the head.

APPETITE AND DIGESTION
- The patient dislikes warm food and likes cold food.
- Colicky pains in the stomach are eased by warm applications.
- Bowel movements are difficult, with sluggish rectal movements leading to "bashful stool" problems.
- Hemorrhoids or anal fissures are extremely painful.

GYNECOLOGICAL PROBLEMS
- There is a history of irregular, difficult, or absent periods.
- Spotting occurs between periods.
- There is a burning, milky-colored vaginal discharge.

JOINTS AND MUSCLES
- Back pains extend from the neck to the base of the spine, are relieved by warmth, and are worse on initial movement after rest.

- Circulation is poor, with a tendency for parts lain on to go numb and to develop "pins and needles."
- Arms and legs feel weak and suffer cramps.

Symptoms are better

- when wrapped up warm;
- when warm compresses are applied;
- in summer weather;
- when lying down.

Symptoms are worse

- in cold, chilly conditions;
- in dry, cold, windy weather;
- with pressure;
- when lying on the painful area;
- during a period.

STAPHYSAGRIA

Key Features

Staphysagria is indicated in the following circumstances.

- There is a marked sensitivity to pains that are sharp, stitching, and stinging in nature.
- Emotional and physical symptoms may be brought on by surgical intervention that is seen to be a violation of privacy or personal integrity: for example, after a hysterectomy or a "high-tech" labor and delivery.
- Physical symptoms emerge as an expression of suppressed anger, rage or indignation.

- The patient is chilly and shivery by nature, and generally emotionally, mentally, and physically oversensitive.

Specific Symptoms

Staphysagria is indicated when the following symptoms occur.

SLEEP

- Drowsiness causes frequent yawning throughout the day, but it is difficult to get to sleep at night.
- When sleep does come, the patient wakes in the morning feeling sulky, unrefreshed, and bad-tempered.

HEADACHE

- Dizziness occurs when lying or sitting down. It is better for getting up and moving about.
- Distracting headaches make thinking difficult, and there are generalized prickling sensations in the head.

APPETITE AND DIGESTION

- An uneasy feeling in the stomach is worse after eating or smoking.
- There is a tight, burning discomfort in the stomach, and queasiness.
- Stomach cramps are brought on by anger and cold drinks.
- Hemorrhoids are distressingly itchy and extremely tender to touch.

CYSTITIS AND KIDNEY PROBLEMS

- Scanty, concentrated, dark-colored urine is passed frequently and urgently.
- Cystitis may be brought on by sexual intercourse, with burning sensations that persist long after the bladder has been emptied.

- Troublesome and irritating sensations are felt, as though a drop of urine is constantly traveling along the urethra.
- Pains are sore, burning, and stinging.
- Chronic cystitis may follow any event that is perceived as a sexual violation or assault.

GYNECOLOGICAL PROBLEMS
- The genital area is extremely sensitive and itchy.
- Residual pain or problems may linger after surgical intervention such as hysterectomy or episiotomy in childbirth. Scars may remain especially sensitive and painful.

JOINTS AND MUSCLES
- Right-sided shoulder pain is much worse for movement.
- Stiff, aching joints are worse for motion and touch.
- Arthritic distortion may affect the appearance of the joints.
- Back pain is worse when at rest and at night.

Symptoms are better

- with warmth;
- after eating;
- when resting (except when suffering from lumbago).

Symptoms are worse

- with emotional upset, anger, or indignation;
- with light touch or pressure;
- during sexual intercourse;
- with smoking;
- in the early morning.

SULPHUR

Key Features

Sulphur is indicated in the following circumstances.

- The patient is intolerant of hot, stuffy conditions and gets very rapidly overheated.
- There may be long-term or recurrent problems with itchy or burning skin eruptions such as eczema, psoriasis, impetigo, and heat rashes.
- She is easily exhausted with a constant need to lie down.
- Itchy skin is much worse for becoming heated in bed at night or after a bath or shower.
- The feet are especially hot and uncomfortable in bed and are often pushed outside the covers to cool down.
- Low blood-sugar levels give rise to weakness, dizziness, and hunger at around 11:00 A.M.
- Skin becomes hot and red very rapidly, especially the areas around the orifices of the body. These include the corners of the mouth, margins of the eyes, and wings of the nose.
- She feels generally much more comfortable for contact with fresh, cool air.
- Discharges such as mucus, pus, or perspiration are often offensive and profuse.

Emotions

Sulphur may be required where the patient:

- is untidy and lives in chaotic surroundings, sometimes starting projects but leaving them half-finished because she has collected too much information to handle;

- is interested in philosophical, abstract issues, and often rambles on at length about simple things;
- becomes introspective and introverted when anxious and depressed and may be obsessional about illness, religious issues, or moral questions;
- has fears that may be linked to poor confidence or low self-esteem and is especially anxious when in bed at night;
- becomes irritable and quarrelsome if criticized, and sulky if challenged;
- alternates between haughtiness and despairing introversion.

Specific Symptoms

Sulphur is indicated when the following symptoms occur.

HOT FLASHES
- Burning flashes of heat are very distressing, and are often brought on by surroundings that are too warm.
- The skin may remain dry and hot during a hot flash, or may be followed by a damp, clammy perspiration that is not localized but affects the body in general.
- Over-heated sensations quickly alternate with chilliness, or some parts of the body may feel flushed while others are chilled.
- Weak, shivery, faint feelings occur before a hot flash.

HEADACHES
- Dizziness can come on at any time, but is especially marked when standing for any substantial time. It is often combined with breathlessness and a sense of weakness and nausea.
- Headaches lodge above the right eye, or may affect the top of the head, which feels over-heated.

- Hot hot flashes accompany a headache.
- Pains are worse from stooping, and when walking out of doors. They are soothed by resting quietly in a moderate, comfortably warm room.
- Weekend and 'holiday' headaches occur as a release from the stresses of the normal week.

APPETITE AND DIGESTION

- Hunger is constant, except at breakfast time.
- Burning indigestion occurs with violent burping.
- Left-sided, colicky pains affect the abdomen with severe distension and swelling.
- The patient craves spicy, sweet, or rich foods. She likes sweet or fatty foods, though they may cause digestive problems and dislikes meat and milk.
- There is urgent, early morning diarrhea that is completely painless.
- Constipation alternates with diarrhea, with small stools that are very difficult to pass.
- Sore, itchy, or burning sensations occur around the anal area at any time, but are especially distressing when getting overheated in bed at night.

CYSTITIS AND KIDNEY PROBLEMS

- Distressing pains in the kidneys with difficulty urinating.
- Frequent desire to pass burning, smarting urine.

GYNECOLOGICAL PROBLEMS

- Periods are irregular, with a flow that stops and starts abruptly.
- Periods are early or late, with dark bleeding that alternates between heavy and scanty amounts.
- Dragging sensations that occur with a prolapse are made worse by standing for a long time.

- Irritation and burning of skin occurs around the entrance to the vagina, alternating with itching and a general sense of discomfort.

JOINTS AND MUSCLES

- The spine is painful and sensitive, with a dislike of the slightest jarring movement or pressure.
- "Dowager's hump" occurs as a result of weakness and lack of tone of the muscles in the spine.
- Joints are stiff and painful and are especially uncomfortable when getting up from a sitting position.
- Limbs frequently "go to sleep" and develop pins and needles when kept in one position for long.
- Pains and cramps are severe at night when becoming warm in bed.

Symptoms are better

- in moderate temperatures;
- in dry, warm weather;
- when lying on the right side;

Symptoms are worse

- with warmth;
- with the heat of the bed;
- when bathing or washing;
- when eating;
- in severely cold conditions;
- when standing or staying for a long time in one position;
- at night;
- midmorning (at around 11:00 A.M.);
- on waking.

Further Reading

GENERAL GUIDES

Castro, Miranda. *The Complete Guide to Homoeopathy: A Guide to Everyday Health Care*. Macmillan, 1990.

Cummings, Dr. Stephen, and Dana Ullman. *Everybody's Guide to Homoeopathic Medicines: Taking Care of Yourself and Your Family with Safe and Effective Medicines*. Gollancz, 1986.

Lockie, Dr. Andrew. *The Family Guide to Homoeopathy: The Safe Form of Medicine for the Future*. Elm Tree Books, 1989.

MacEoin, Beth, *Homoeopathy: Headway Lifeguides*. Headway, 1992.

Ullman, Dana. *Homoeopathy, Medicine for the Twenty-First Century*. Thorsons, 1989.

Weiner, Michael, and Kathleen Goss. *The Complete Book of Homeopathy*. Bantam, 1982.

ALTERNATIVE MEDICINE AND WOMEN'S HEALTH

Handley, Rima. *Homoeopathy for Women*. Thorsons, 1993.

Lockie, Dr. Andrew, and Dr. Nicola Geddes. *The Woman's Guide to Homoeopathy: The Natural Way to a Healthier Life for Women*. Hamish Hamilton, 1992.

MacEoin, Beth. *Healthy by Nature: A Woman's Guide to Positive Health and Vitality in a Stressful World.* Thorsons, 1994.

MacEoin, Beth. *Homoeopathy for Women: A Guide to Vital Health.* Headway, 1995.

Scott, Julian and Susan. *Natural Medicine for Women: Drug-free Healthcare for Women of All Ages.* Gaia, 1991.

Westcott, Patsy. *Alternative Health Care for Women: A Compendium of Natural Approaches to Women's Health and Well-being.* Grapevine, 1987.

GENERAL GUIDES FOR WOMEN

Bradford, Nikki. *The Well Woman's Self-Help Directory.* Sidgwick and Jackson, 1990.

Llewellyn-Jones, Derek. *Everywoman: A Gynaecological Guide for Life.* Penguin, 1993.

Phillips, Angela, and Jill Rakusen. *The New Our Bodies Ourselves: A Health Book For and By Women.* Penguin, 1989.

Stoppard, Dr. Miriam. *Every Woman's Lifeguide: How to Achieve and Maintain Fitness, Health, and Happiness in Today's World.* Optima, 1988.

MENOPAUSE

Dickson, Anne, and Nikki Henriques. *Menopause: The Woman's View.* Grapevine, 1987.

Kahn, Ada, and Linda Hughey Holt. *Menopause: The Best Years of Your Life.* Bloomsbury, 1993.

Sheehy, Gail. *The Silent Passage: Menopause.* HarperCollins, 1991.

Stoppard, Dr Miriam. *Menopause: The Complete Practical Guide to Managing Your Life and Maintaining Physical and Emotional Well-being.* Dorling Kindersley, 1994.

HORMONE REPLACEMENT THERAPY

Bawdon, Fiona. "HRT: The Myths Exploded," *What Doctors Don't Tell You* 4, no. 9 (1994).

Nicol, Rosemary. *Everything You Need to Know about Osteoporosis.* Sheldon Press, 1990.

Nicol, Rosemary. *Hormone Replacement Therapy: Your Guide to Making an Informed Choice.* Vermillion, 1993.

~

Resources

Boiron/Borneman
6 Campus Boulevard
Building A
Newtown Square, PA 19073
(610) 325-7464 or 800-BOIRON-1
West Coast Branch:
98C West Cochran Street
Simi Valley, CA 93065
(805) 582-9091 or 800-BOIRON-1

Manufacturer of homeopathic remedies.

Homeopathic Educational Services
2124 Kittredge Street
Berkeley, CA 94704
(510) 649-0294 or 800-359-9051 (orders only)

Extensive list of books on homeopathy and related health issues; remedy kits. Free catalog.

Homeopathy Online: A Journal of Homeopathic Medicine
www.lyghtforce.com/HomeopathyOnline

Journal on the worldwide web. (Other homeopathy-related Web sites exist, but addresses change rapidly. Use a search engine to find the latest sites.)

International Foundation for Homeopathy (IFH)
P.O. Box 7
Edmonds, WA 98020
(206) 776-4147; fax: 206-776-1499

A nonprofit organization dedicated to the education of professional homeopaths according to the highest standards of classical homeopathy. Activities include professional courses, an annual conference, and a bimonthly magazine. Referrals to graduates of the (IFH) professional course will be provided with a SASE.

National Center for Homeopathy (NCH)
801 North Fairfax Street
Suite 306
Alexandria, VA 22314
(703) 548-7790; fax: 703-548-7792
nchinfo@igc.apc.org

A nonprofit membership organization dedicated to promoting homeopathy in the U.S. through education, publication, research, and membership services. Membership is $40/year and includes the monthly magazine *Homeopathy Today* and the annual directory of practitioners, study groups, and resources. The directory lists licensed health-care professionals who devote 25 to 100 percent of their practice to homeopathy. An information packet, which includes the directory, is available to nonmembers for $6. The directory is also available at http://www.healthy.net/nch.

Standard Homeopathic Company
154 West 131 Street
Box 61067
Los Angeles, CA 90061
(800) 624-9659 or (213) 321-4284

Manufacturer of a full line of homeopathic medicines in various dosage forms, including tincture, dilution, pellets, and tablets.

Index